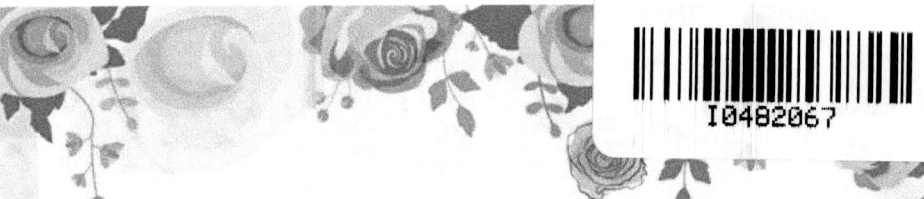

VISIT TO THE DOCTOR

Belong to ..

Name ....

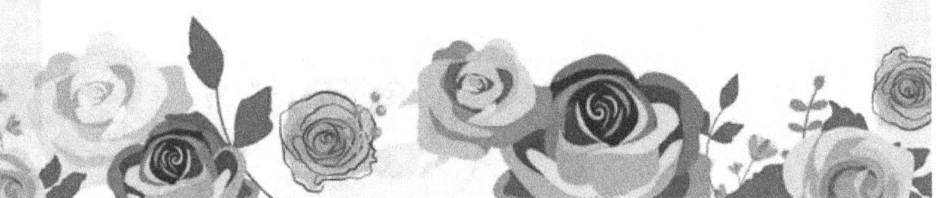

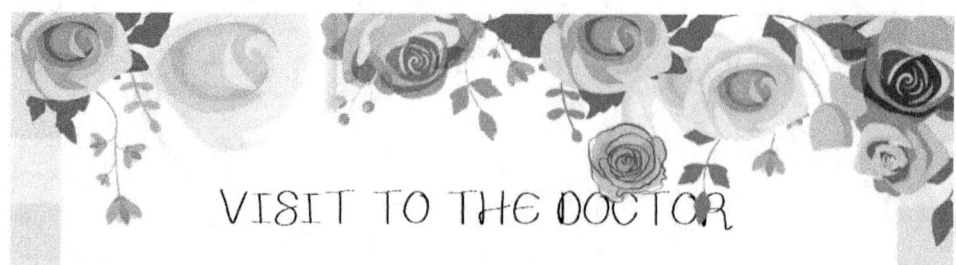

VISIT TO THE DOCTOR

Date	
Doctor	
Hospital or Clinic	
Reason for Visit	
Diasnosis	
Doctor's Comment & Notes	
Follow Up	

Date	
Doctor	
Hospital or Clinic	
Reason for Visit	
Diasnosis	
Doctor,s Comment & Notes	
Follow Up	

Date	
Doctor	
Hospital or Clinic	
Reason for Visit	
Diasnosis	
Doctor's Comment & Notes	
Follow Up	

Date	
Doctor	
Hospital or Clinic	
Reason for Visit	
Diasnosis	
Doctor's Comment & Notes	
Follow Up	

Notes:

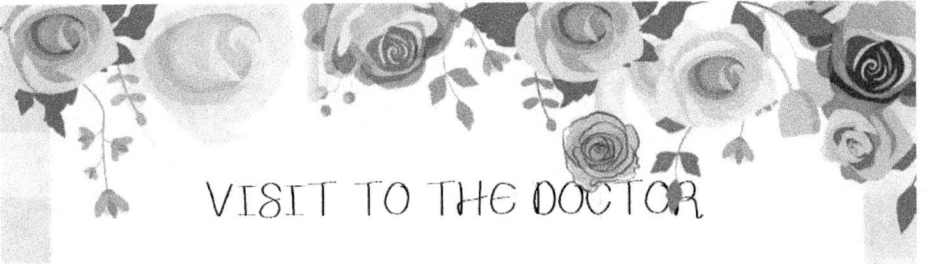

VISIT TO THE DOCTOR

Date	
Doctor	
Hospital or Clinic	
Reason for Visit	
Diasnosis	
Doctor's Comment & Notes	
Follow Up	

Date	
Doctor	
Hospital or Clinic	
Reason for Visit	
Diasnosis	
Doctor,s Comment & Notes	
Follow Up	

Date	
Doctor	
Hospital or Clinic	
Reason for Visit	
Diasnosis	
Doctor's Comment & Notes	
Follow Up	

Date	
Doctor	
Hospital or Clinic	
Reason for Visit	
Diasnosis	
Doctor's Comment & Notes	
Follow Up	

Notes:

_____

_____

_____

_____

_____

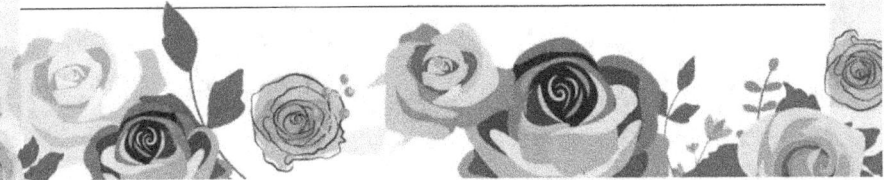

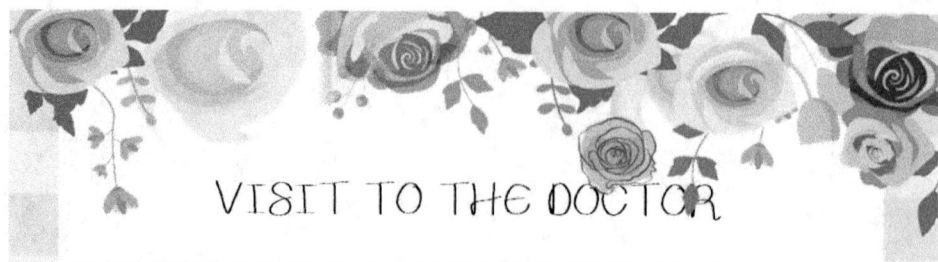

VISIT TO THE DOCTOR

Date		Date	
Doctor		Doctor	
Hospital or Clinic		Hospital or Clinic	
Reason for Visit		Reason for Visit	
Diasnosis		Diasnosis	
Doctor's Comment & Notes		Doctor,s Comment & Notes	
Follow Up		Follow Up	

Date		Date	
Doctor		Doctor	
Hospital or Clinic		Hospital or Clinic	
Reason for Visit		Reason for Visit	
Diasnosis		Diasnosis	
Doctor's Comment & Notes		Doctor's Comment & Notes	
Follow Up		Follow Up	

Notes:

_____

_____

_____

_____

_____

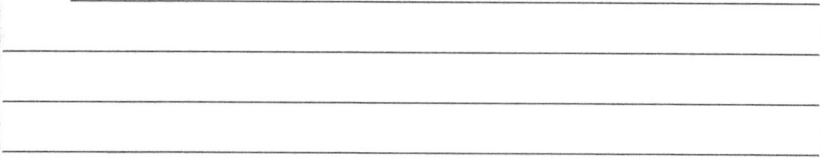

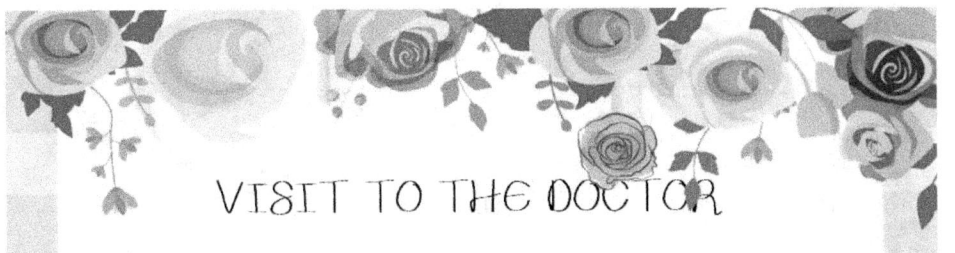

VISIT TO THE DOCTOR

Date			Date	
Doctor			Doctor	
Hospital or Clinic			Hospital or Clinic	
Reason for Visit			Reason for Visit	
Diasnosis			Diasnosis	
Doctor's Comment & Notes			Doctor,s Comment & Notes	
Follow Up			Follow Up	

Date			Date	
Doctor			Doctor	
Hospital or Clinic			Hospital or Clinic	
Reason for Visit			Reason for Visit	
Diasnosis			Diasnosis	
Doctor's Comment & Notes			Doctor's Comment & Notes	
Follow Up			Follow Up	

Notes: _____

_____

_____

_____

_____

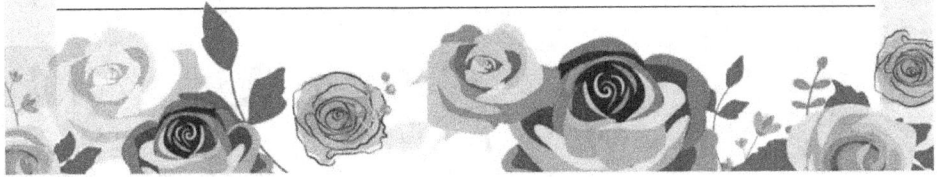

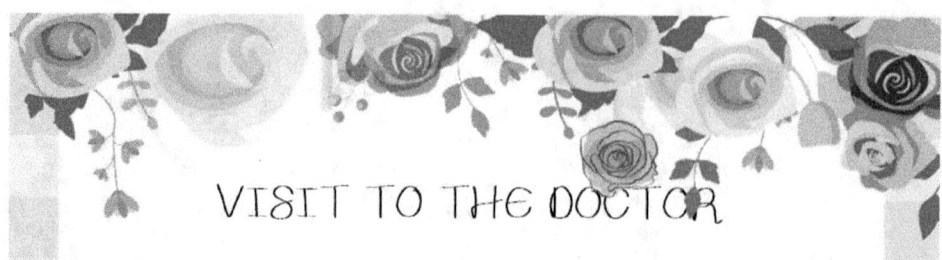

VISIT TO THE DOCTOR

Date			Date	
Doctor			Doctor	
Hospital or Clinic			Hospital or Clinic	
Reason for Visit			Reason for Visit	
Diasnosis			Diasnosis	
Doctor's Comment & Notes			Doctor,s Comment & Notes	
Follow Up			Follow Up	

Date			Date	
Doctor			Doctor	
Hospital or Clinic			Hospital or Clinic	
Reason for Visit			Reason for Visit	
Diasnosis			Diasnosis	
Doctor's Comment & Notes			Doctor's Comment & Notes	
Follow Up			Follow Up	

Notes: _____

_____

_____

_____

_____

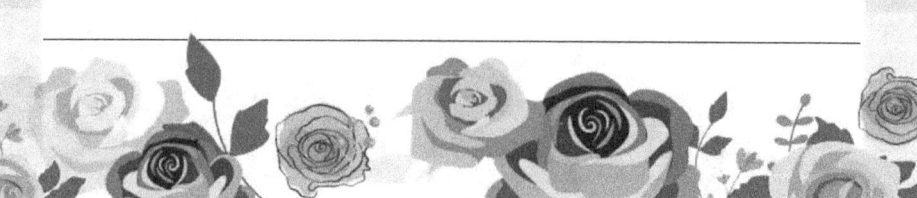

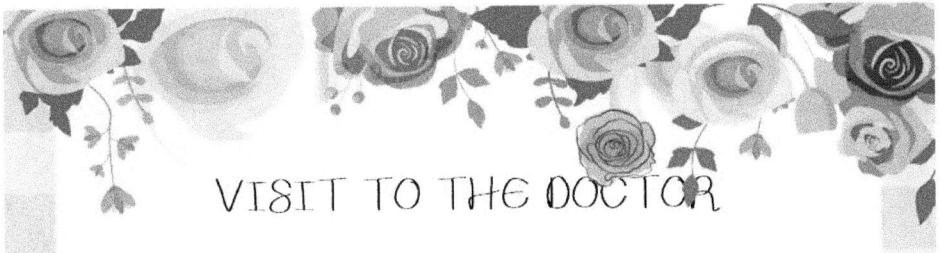

VISIT TO THE DOCTOR

Date	
Doctor	
Hospital or Clinic	
Reason for Visit	
Diasnosis	
Doctor's Comment & Notes	
Follow Up	

Date	
Doctor	
Hospital or Clinic	
Reason for Visit	
Diasnosis	
Doctor,s Comment & Notes	
Follow Up	

Date	
Doctor	
Hospital or Clinic	
Reason for Visit	
Diasnosis	
Doctor's Comment & Notes	
Follow Up	

Date	
Doctor	
Hospital or Clinic	
Reason for Visit	
Diasnosis	
Doctor's Comment & Notes	
Follow Up	

Notes:
_____
_____
_____
_____
_____
_____

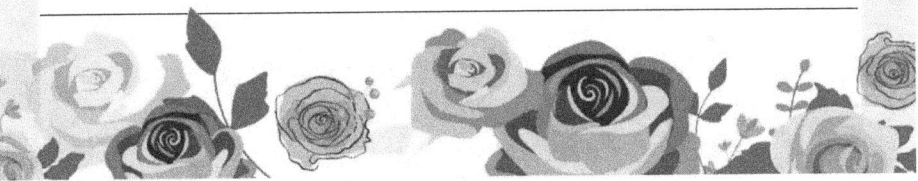

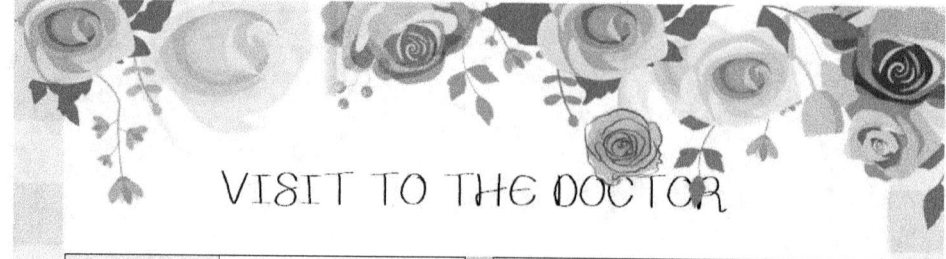

VISIT TO THE DOCTOR

Date	
Doctor	
Hospital or Clinic	
Reason for Visit	
Diasnosis	
Doctor's Comment & Notes	
Follow Up	

Date	
Doctor	
Hospital or Clinic	
Reason for Visit	
Diasnosis	
Doctor,s Comment & Notes	
Follow Up	

Date	
Doctor	
Hospital or Clinic	
Reason for Visit	
Diasnosis	
Doctor's Comment & Notes	
Follow Up	

Date	
Doctor	
Hospital or Clinic	
Reason for Visit	
Diasnosis	
Doctor's Comment & Notes	
Follow Up	

Notes:

_____

_____

_____

_____

_____

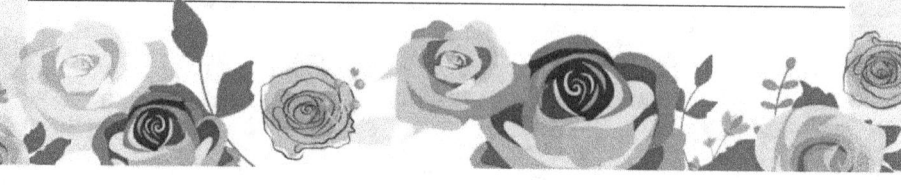

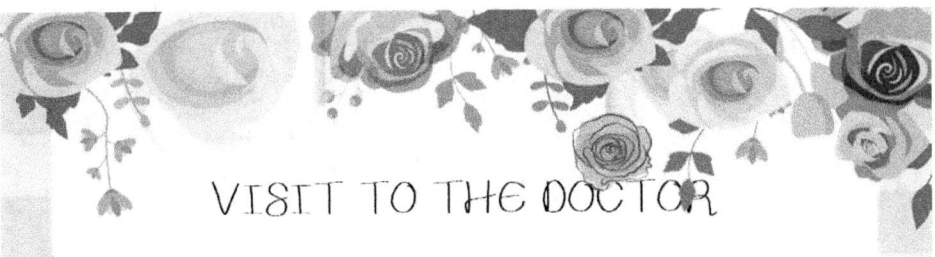

VISIT TO THE DOCTOR

Date		Date	
Doctor		Doctor	
Hospital or Clinic		Hospital or Clinic	
Reason for Visit		Reason for Visit	
Diasnosis		Diasnosis	
Doctor's Comment & Notes		Doctor,s Comment & Notes	
Follow Up		Follow Up	

Date		Date	
Doctor		Doctor	
Hospital or Clinic		Hospital or Clinic	
Reason for Visit		Reason for Visit	
Diasnosis		Diasnosis	
Doctor's Comment & Notes		Doctor's Comment & Notes	
Follow Up		Follow Up	

Notes:

_____

_____

_____

_____

_____

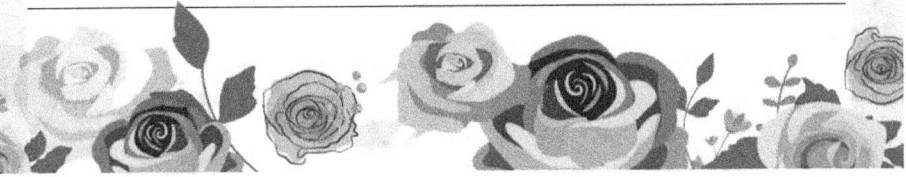

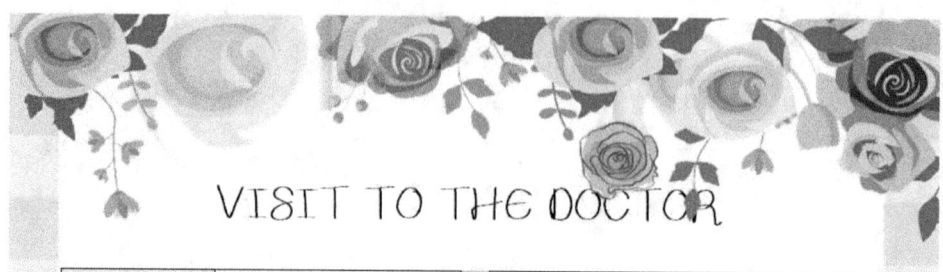

VISIT TO THE DOCTOR

Date	
Doctor	
Hospital or Clinic	
Reason for Visit	
Diasnosis	
Doctor's Comment & Notes	
Follow Up	

Date	
Doctor	
Hospital or Clinic	
Reason for Visit	
Diasnosis	
Doctor,s Comment & Notes	
Follow Up	

Date	
Doctor	
Hospital or Clinic	
Reason for Visit	
Diasnosis	
Doctor's Comment & Notes	
Follow Up	

Date	
Doctor	
Hospital or Clinic	
Reason for Visit	
Diasnosis	
Doctor's Comment & Notes	
Follow Up	

Notes:

_____

_____

_____

_____

_____

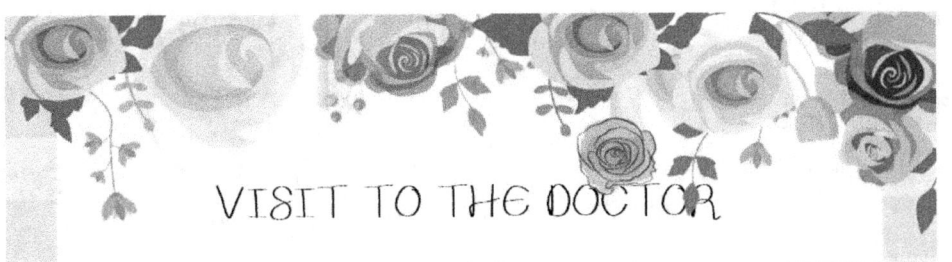

VISIT TO THE DOCTOR

Date	
Doctor	
Hospital or Clinic	
Reason for Visit	
Diasnosis	
Doctor's Comment & Notes	
Follow Up	

Date	
Doctor	
Hospital or Clinic	
Reason for Visit	
Diasnosis	
Doctor,s Comment & Notes	
Follow Up	

Date	
Doctor	
Hospital or Clinic	
Reason for Visit	
Diasnosis	
Doctor's Comment & Notes	
Follow Up	

Date	
Doctor	
Hospital or Clinic	
Reason for Visit	
Diasnosis	
Doctor's Comment & Notes	
Follow Up	

Notes:

_____

_____

_____

_____

_____

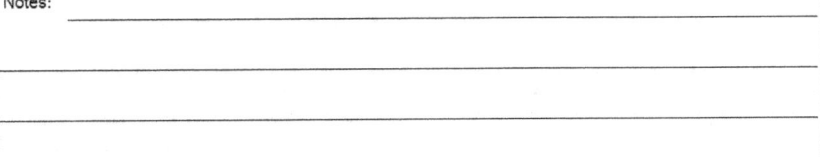

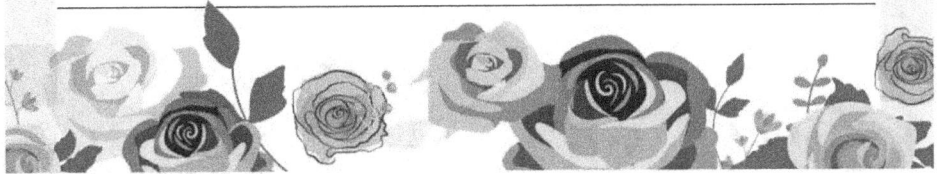

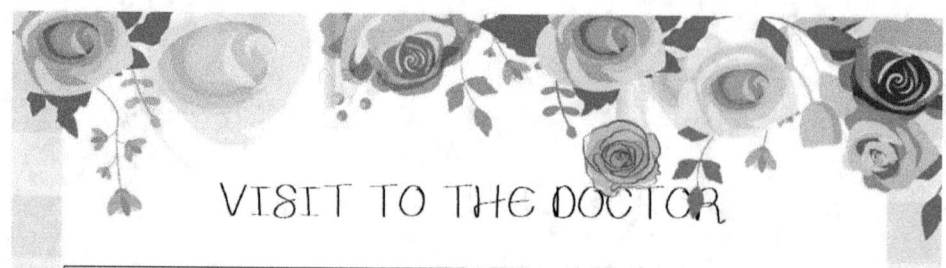

VISIT TO THE DOCTOR

Date	
Doctor	
Hospital or Clinic	
Reason for Visit	
Diasnosis	
Doctor's Comment & Notes	
Follow Up	

Date	
Doctor	
Hospital or Clinic	
Reason for Visit	
Diasnosis	
Doctor,s Comment & Notes	
Follow Up	

Date	
Doctor	
Hospital or Clinic	
Reason for Visit	
Diasnosis	
Doctor's Comment & Notes	
Follow Up	

Date	
Doctor	
Hospital or Clinic	
Reason for Visit	
Diasnosis	
Doctor's Comment & Notes	
Follow Up	

Notes:

_____

_____

_____

_____

_____

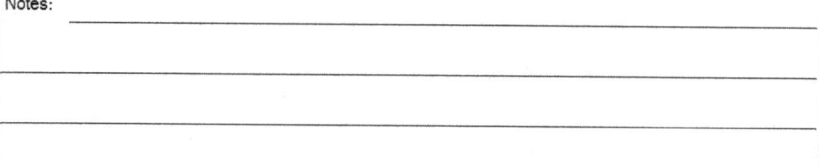

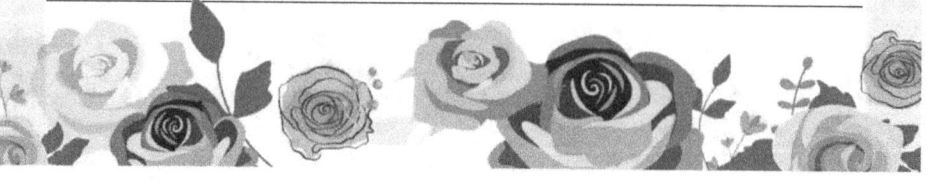

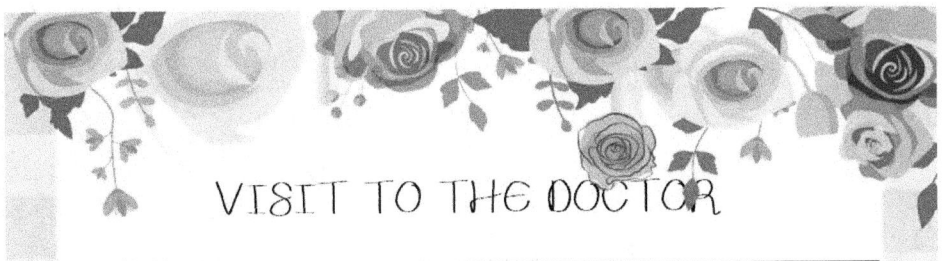

VISIT TO THE DOCTOR

Date	
Doctor	
Hospital or Clinic	
Reason for Visit	
Diasnosis	
Doctor's Comment & Notes	
Follow Up	

Date	
Doctor	
Hospital or Clinic	
Reason for Visit	
Diasnosis	
Doctor,s Comment & Notes	
Follow Up	

Date	
Doctor	
Hospital or Clinic	
Reason for Visit	
Diasnosis	
Doctor's Comment & Notes	
Follow Up	

Date	
Doctor	
Hospital or Clinic	
Reason for Visit	
Diasnosis	
Doctor's Comment & Notes	
Follow Up	

Notes:

_____

_____

_____

_____

_____

_____

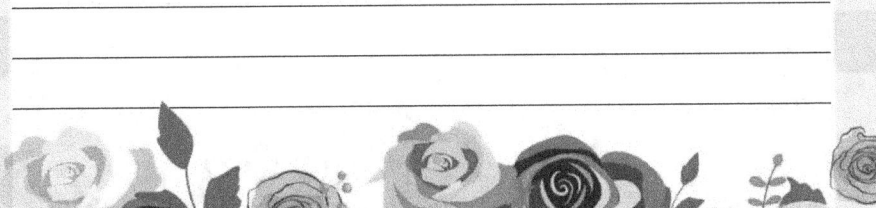

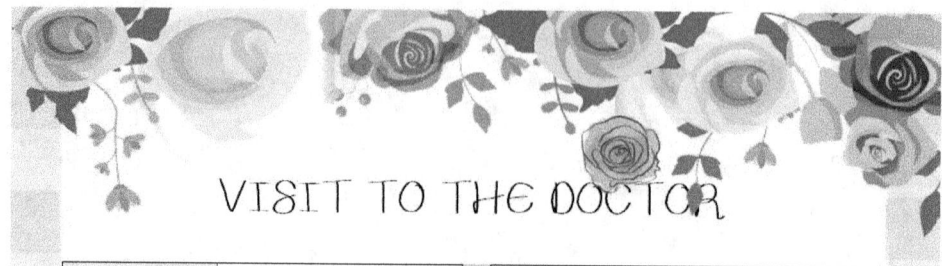

VISIT TO THE DOCTOR

Date	
Doctor	
Hospital or Clinic	
Reason for Visit	
Diasnosis	
Doctor's Comment & Notes	
Follow Up	

Date	
Doctor	
Hospital or Clinic	
Reason for Visit	
Diasnosis	
Doctor,s Comment & Notes	
Follow Up	

Date	
Doctor	
Hospital or Clinic	
Reason for Visit	
Diasnosis	
Doctor's Comment & Notes	
Follow Up	

Date	
Doctor	
Hospital or Clinic	
Reason for Visit	
Diasnosis	
Doctor's Comment & Notes	
Follow Up	

Notes:

_____

_____

_____

_____

_____

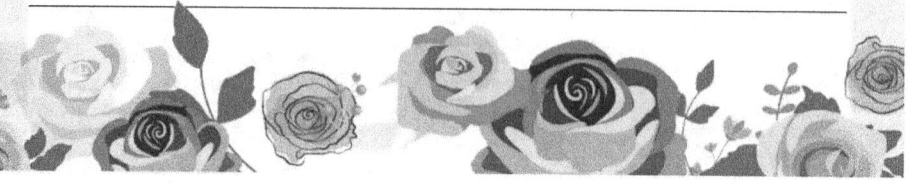

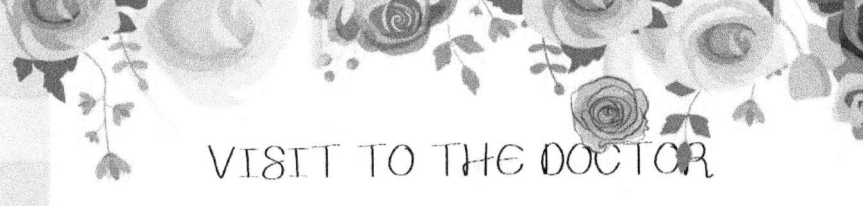

VISIT TO THE DOCTOR

Date	
Doctor	
Hospital or Clinic	
Reason for Visit	
Diasnosis	
Doctor's Comment & Notes	
Follow Up	

Date	
Doctor	
Hospital or Clinic	
Reason for Visit	
Diasnosis	
Doctor,s Comment & Notes	
Follow Up	

Date	
Doctor	
Hospital or Clinic	
Reason for Visit	
Diasnosis	
Doctor's Comment & Notes	
Follow Up	

Date	
Doctor	
Hospital or Clinic	
Reason for Visit	
Diasnosis	
Doctor's Comment & Notes	
Follow Up	

Notes:
_____
_____
_____
_____
_____

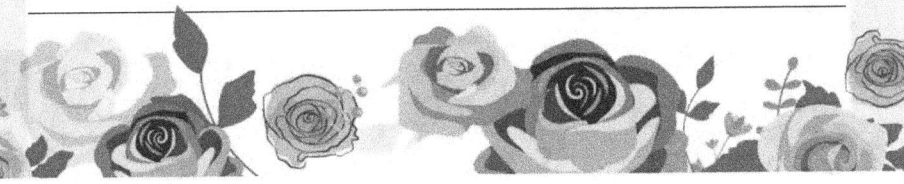

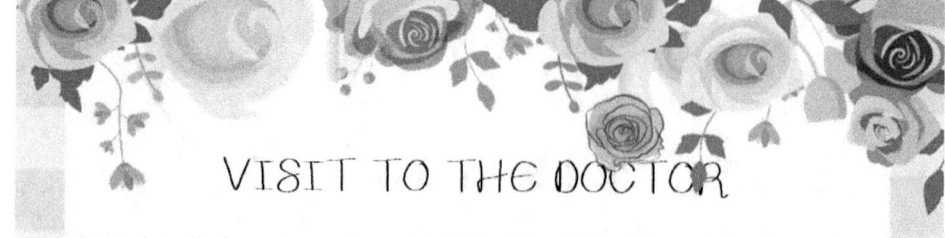

VISIT TO THE DOCTOR

Date	
Doctor	
Hospital or Clinic	
Reason for Visit	
Diasnosis	
Doctor's Comment & Notes	
Follow Up	

Date	
Doctor	
Hospital or Clinic	
Reason for Visit	
Diasnosis	
Doctor,s Comment & Notes	
Follow Up	

Date	
Doctor	
Hospital or Clinic	
Reason for Visit	
Diasnosis	
Doctor's Comment & Notes	
Follow Up	

Date	
Doctor	
Hospital or Clinic	
Reason for Visit	
Diasnosis	
Doctor's Comment & Notes	
Follow Up	

Notes:

_____

_____

_____

_____

_____

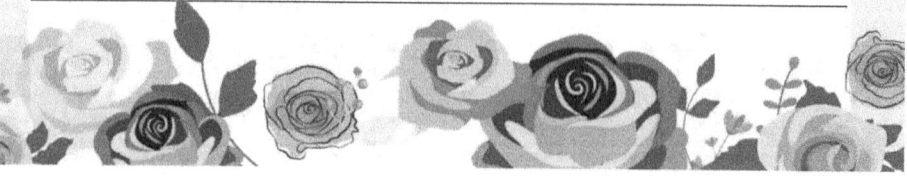

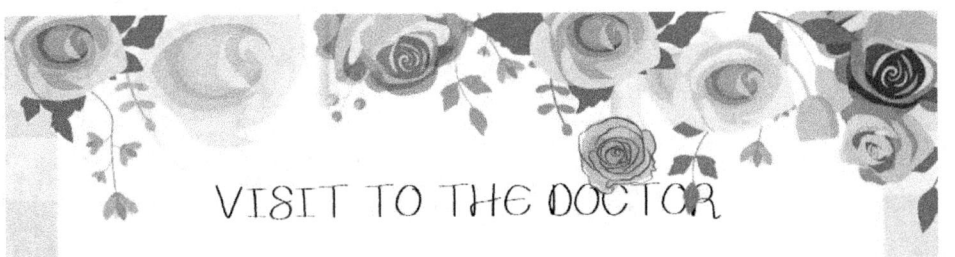

VISIT TO THE DOCTOR

Date	
Doctor	
Hospital or Clinic	
Reason for Visit	
Diasnosis	
Doctor's Comment & Notes	
Follow Up	

Date	
Doctor	
Hospital or Clinic	
Reason for Visit	
Diasnosis	
Doctor,s Comment & Notes	
Follow Up	

Date	
Doctor	
Hospital or Clinic	
Reason for Visit	
Diasnosis	
Doctor's Comment & Notes	
Follow Up	

Date	
Doctor	
Hospital or Clinic	
Reason for Visit	
Diasnosis	
Doctor's Comment & Notes	
Follow Up	

Notes: _____

_____

_____

_____

_____

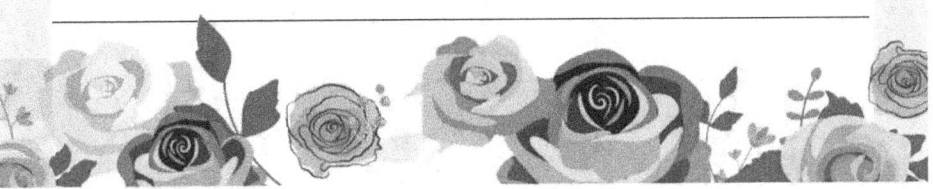

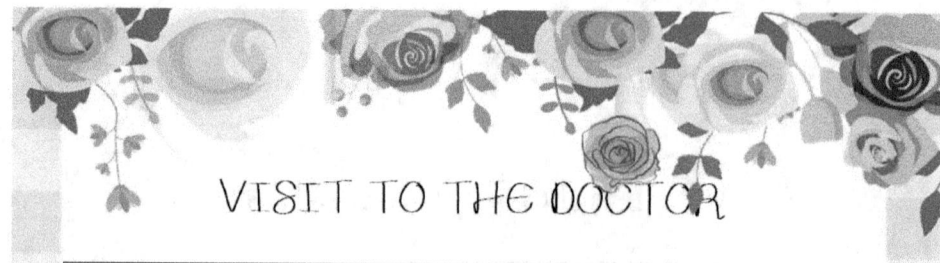

VISIT TO THE DOCTOR

Date	
Doctor	
Hospital or Clinic	
Reason for Visit	
Diasnosis	
Doctor's Comment & Notes	
Follow Up	

Date	
Doctor	
Hospital or Clinic	
Reason for Visit	
Diasnosis	
Doctor,s Comment & Notes	
Follow Up	

Date	
Doctor	
Hospital or Clinic	
Reason for Visit	
Diasnosis	
Doctor's Comment & Notes	
Follow Up	

Date	
Doctor	
Hospital or Clinic	
Reason for Visit	
Diasnosis	
Doctor's Comment & Notes	
Follow Up	

Notes:

_____

_____

_____

_____

_____

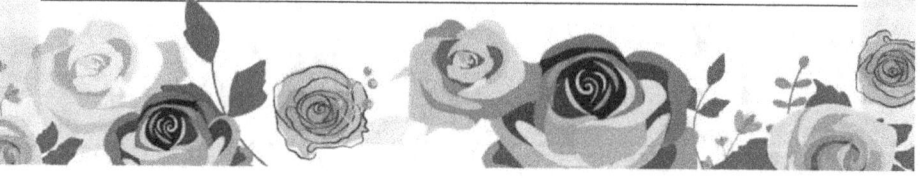

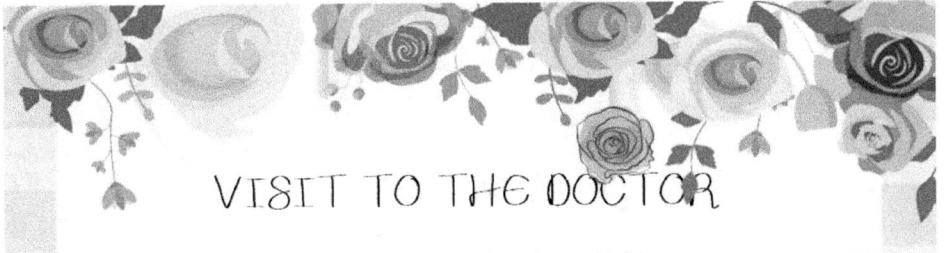

VISIT TO THE DOCTOR

Date	
Doctor	
Hospital or Clinic	
Reason for Visit	
Diasnosis	
Doctor's Comment & Notes	
Follow Up	

Date	
Doctor	
Hospital or Clinic	
Reason for Visit	
Diasnosis	
Doctor,s Comment & Notes	
Follow Up	

Date	
Doctor	
Hospital or Clinic	
Reason for Visit	
Diasnosis	
Doctor's Comment & Notes	
Follow Up	

Date	
Doctor	
Hospital or Clinic	
Reason for Visit	
Diasnosis	
Doctor's Comment & Notes	
Follow Up	

Notes:

_____

_____

_____

_____

_____

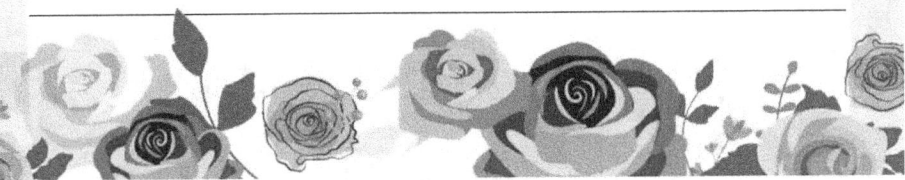

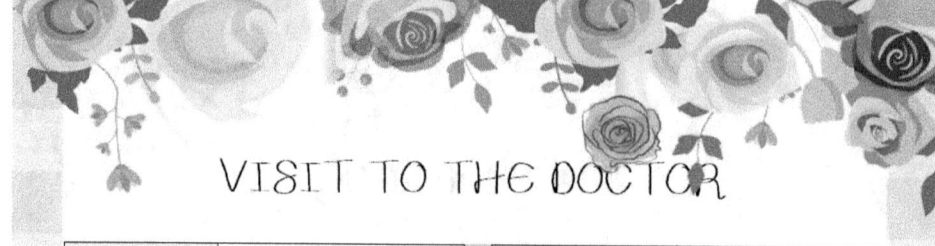

VISIT TO THE DOCTOR

Date	
Doctor	
Hospital or Clinic	
Reason for Visit	
Diasnosis	
Doctor's Comment & Notes	
Follow Up	

Date	
Doctor	
Hospital or Clinic	
Reason for Visit	
Diasnosis	
Doctor,s Comment & Notes	
Follow Up	

Date	
Doctor	
Hospital or Clinic	
Reason for Visit	
Diasnosis	
Doctor's Comment & Notes	
Follow Up	

Date	
Doctor	
Hospital or Clinic	
Reason for Visit	
Diasnosis	
Doctor's Comment & Notes	
Follow Up	

Notes:

_____

_____

_____

_____

_____

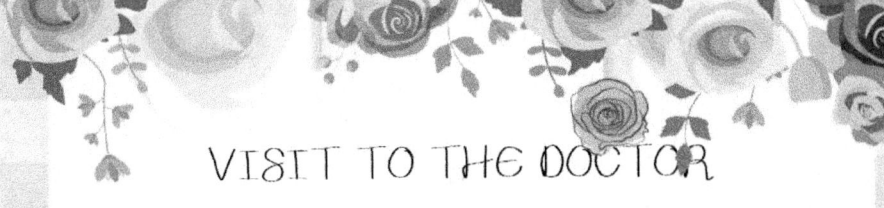

VISIT TO THE DOCTOR

Date	
Doctor	
Hospital or Clinic	
Reason for Visit	
Diasnosis	
Doctor's Comment & Notes	
Follow Up	

Date	
Doctor	
Hospital or Clinic	
Reason for Visit	
Diasnosis	
Doctor,s Comment & Notes	
Follow Up	

Date	
Doctor	
Hospital or Clinic	
Reason for Visit	
Diasnosis	
Doctor's Comment & Notes	
Follow Up	

Date	
Doctor	
Hospital or Clinic	
Reason for Visit	
Diasnosis	
Doctor's Comment & Notes	
Follow Up	

Notes:

_____

_____

_____

_____

_____

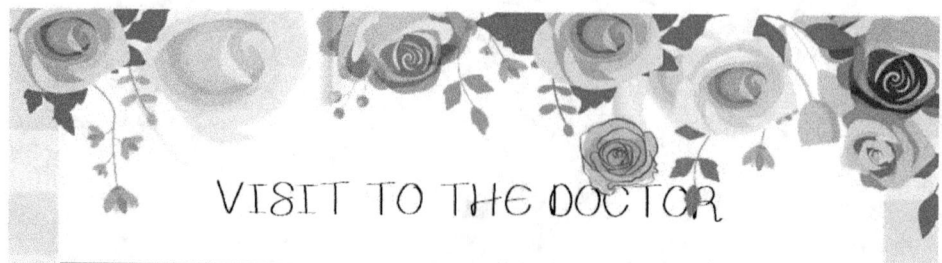

VISIT TO THE DOCTOR

Date	
Doctor	
Hospital or Clinic	
Reason for Visit	
Diasnosis	
Doctor's Comment & Notes	
Follow Up	

Date	
Doctor	
Hospital or Clinic	
Reason for Visit	
Diasnosis	
Doctor,s Comment & Notes	
Follow Up	

Date	
Doctor	
Hospital or Clinic	
Reason for Visit	
Diasnosis	
Doctor's Comment & Notes	
Follow Up	

Date	
Doctor	
Hospital or Clinic	
Reason for Visit	
Diasnosis	
Doctor's Comment & Notes	
Follow Up	

Notes:

_____

_____

_____

_____

_____

_____

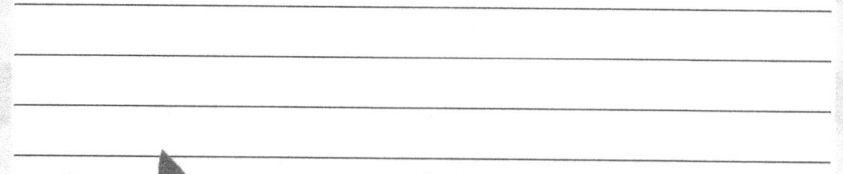

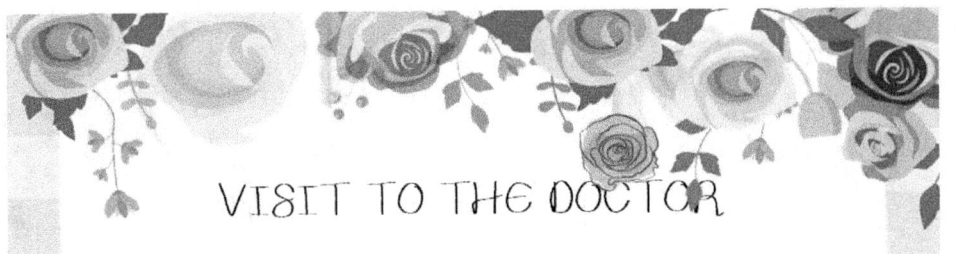

VISIT TO THE DOCTOR

Date	
Doctor	
Hospital or Clinic	
Reason for Visit	
Diasnosis	
Doctor's Comment & Notes	
Follow Up	

Date	
Doctor	
Hospital or Clinic	
Reason for Visit	
Diasnosis	
Doctor,s Comment & Notes	
Follow Up	

Date	
Doctor	
Hospital or Clinic	
Reason for Visit	
Diasnosis	
Doctor's Comment & Notes	
Follow Up	

Date	
Doctor	
Hospital or Clinic	
Reason for Visit	
Diasnosis	
Doctor's Comment & Notes	
Follow Up	

Notes:

_____

_____

_____

_____

_____

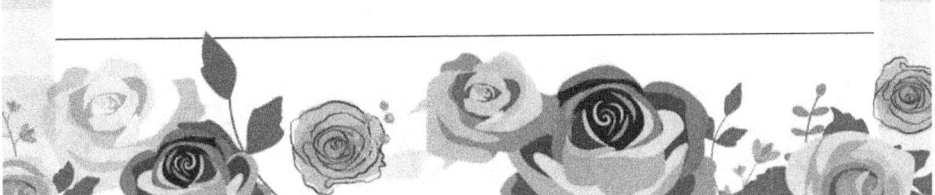

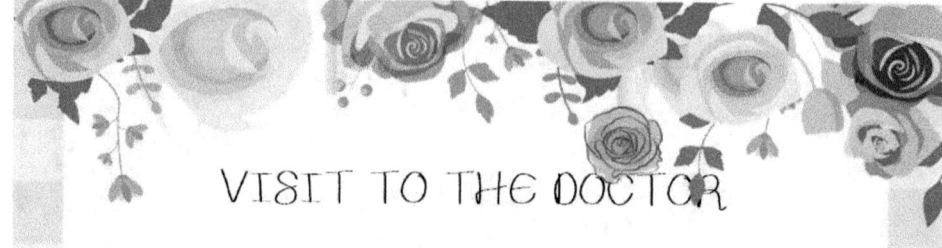

VISIT TO THE DOCTOR

Date	
Doctor	
Hospital or Clinic	
Reason for Visit	
Diasnosis	
Doctor's Comment & Notes	
Follow Up	

Date	
Doctor	
Hospital or Clinic	
Reason for Visit	
Diasnosis	
Doctor,s Comment & Notes	
Follow Up	

Date	
Doctor	
Hospital or Clinic	
Reason for Visit	
Diasnosis	
Doctor's Comment & Notes	
Follow Up	

Date	
Doctor	
Hospital or Clinic	
Reason for Visit	
Diasnosis	
Doctor's Comment & Notes	
Follow Up	

Notes:

_____

_____

_____

_____

_____

_____

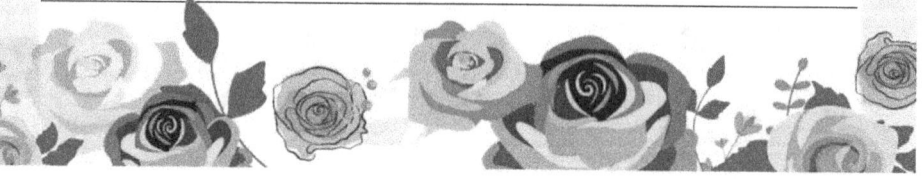

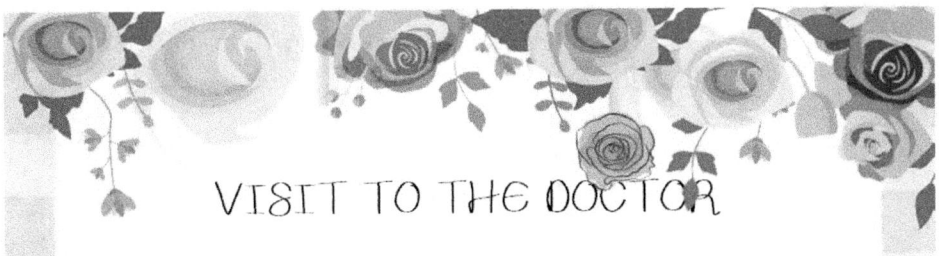

VISIT TO THE DOCTOR

Date	
Doctor	
Hospital or Clinic	
Reason for Visit	
Diasnosis	
Doctor's Comment & Notes	
Follow Up	

Date	
Doctor	
Hospital or Clinic	
Reason for Visit	
Diasnosis	
Doctor,s Comment & Notes	
Follow Up	

Date	
Doctor	
Hospital or Clinic	
Reason for Visit	
Diasnosis	
Doctor's Comment & Notes	
Follow Up	

Date	
Doctor	
Hospital or Clinic	
Reason for Visit	
Diasnosis	
Doctor's Comment & Notes	
Follow Up	

Notes: _____

_____

_____

_____

_____

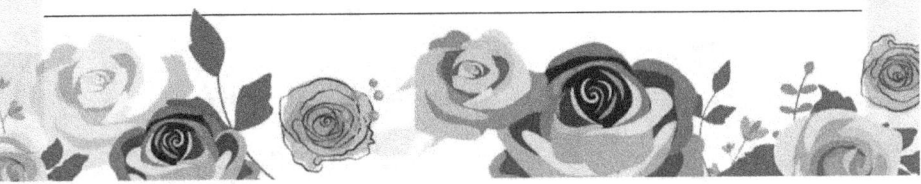

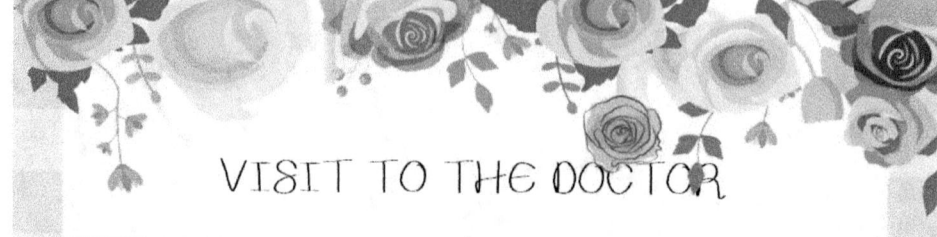

VISIT TO THE DOCTOR

Date	
Doctor	
Hospital or Clinic	
Reason for Visit	
Diasnosis	
Doctor's Comment & Notes	
Follow Up	

Date	
Doctor	
Hospital or Clinic	
Reason for Visit	
Diasnosis	
Doctor,s Comment & Notes	
Follow Up	

Date	
Doctor	
Hospital or Clinic	
Reason for Visit	
Diasnosis	
Doctor's Comment & Notes	
Follow Up	

Date	
Doctor	
Hospital or Clinic	
Reason for Visit	
Diasnosis	
Doctor's Comment & Notes	
Follow Up	

Notes:

_____

_____

_____

_____

_____

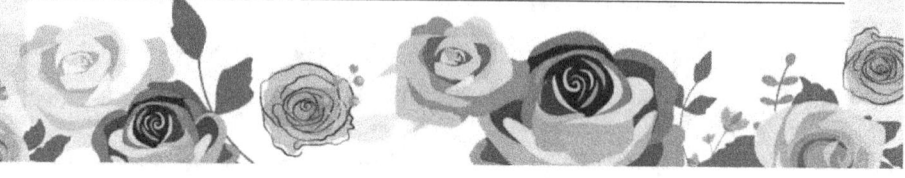

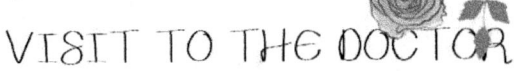

VISIT TO THE DOCTOR

Date	
Doctor	
Hospital or Clinic	
Reason for Visit	
Diasnosis	
Doctor's Comment & Notes	
Follow Up	

Date	
Doctor	
Hospital or Clinic	
Reason for Visit	
Diasnosis	
Doctor,s Comment & Notes	
Follow Up	

Date	
Doctor	
Hospital or Clinic	
Reason for Visit	
Diasnosis	
Doctor's Comment & Notes	
Follow Up	

Date	
Doctor	
Hospital or Clinic	
Reason for Visit	
Diasnosis	
Doctor's Comment & Notes	
Follow Up	

Notes:

_____

_____

_____

_____

_____

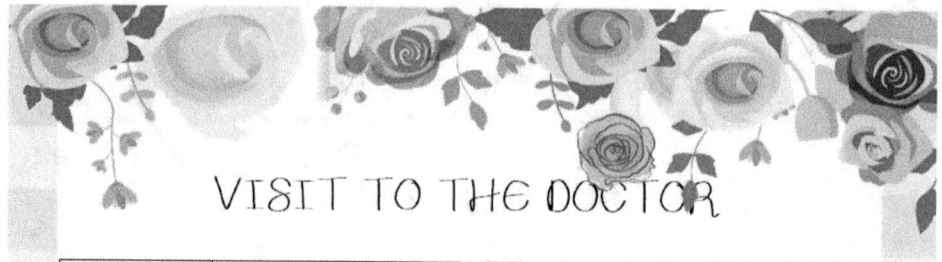

VISIT TO THE DOCTOR

Date	
Doctor	
Hospital or Clinic	
Reason for Visit	
Diasnosis	
Doctor's Comment & Notes	
Follow Up	

Date	
Doctor	
Hospital or Clinic	
Reason for Visit	
Diasnosis	
Doctor,s Comment & Notes	
Follow Up	

Date	
Doctor	
Hospital or Clinic	
Reason for Visit	
Diasnosis	
Doctor's Comment & Notes	
Follow Up	

Date	
Doctor	
Hospital or Clinic	
Reason for Visit	
Diasnosis	
Doctor's Comment & Notes	
Follow Up	

Notes:

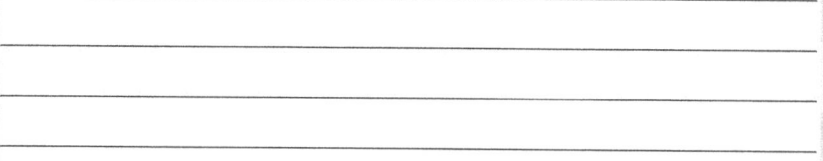

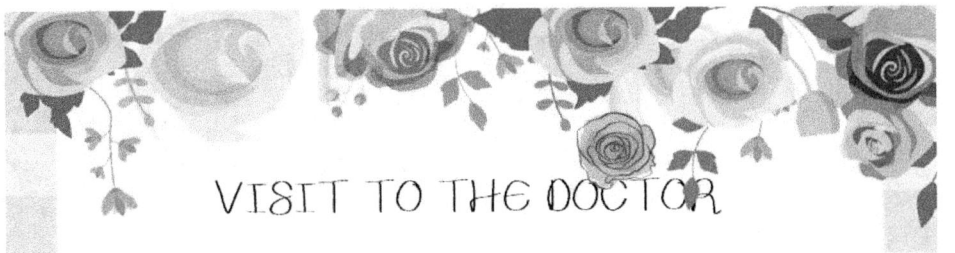

VISIT TO THE DOCTOR

Date	
Doctor	
Hospital or Clinic	
Reason for Visit	
Diasnosis	
Doctor's Comment & Notes	
Follow Up	

Date	
Doctor	
Hospital or Clinic	
Reason for Visit	
Diasnosis	
Doctor,s Comment & Notes	
Follow Up	

Date	
Doctor	
Hospital or Clinic	
Reason for Visit	
Diasnosis	
Doctor's Comment & Notes	
Follow Up	

Date	
Doctor	
Hospital or Clinic	
Reason for Visit	
Diasnosis	
Doctor's Comment & Notes	
Follow Up	

Notes: _____

_____

_____

_____

_____

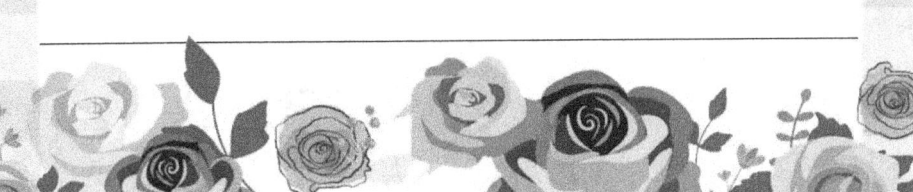

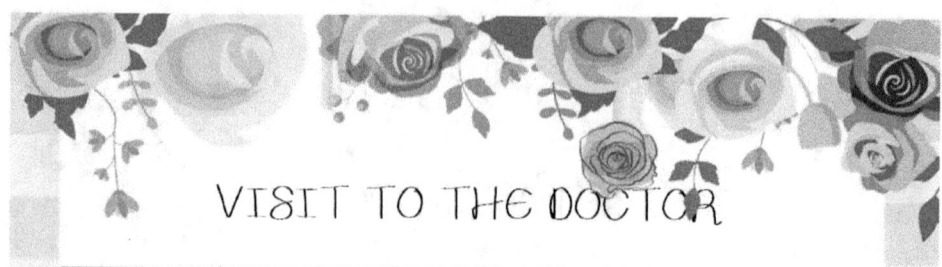

VISIT TO THE DOCTOR

Date			Date	
Doctor			Doctor	
Hospital or Clinic			Hospital or Clinic	
Reason for Visit			Reason for Visit	
Diasnosis			Diasnosis	
Doctor's Comment & Notes			Doctor,s Comment & Notes	
Follow Up			Follow Up	

Date			Date	
Doctor			Doctor	
Hospital or Clinic			Hospital or Clinic	
Reason for Visit			Reason for Visit	
Diasnosis			Diasnosis	
Doctor's Comment & Notes			Doctor's Comment & Notes	
Follow Up			Follow Up	

Notes:

_____

_____

_____

_____

_____

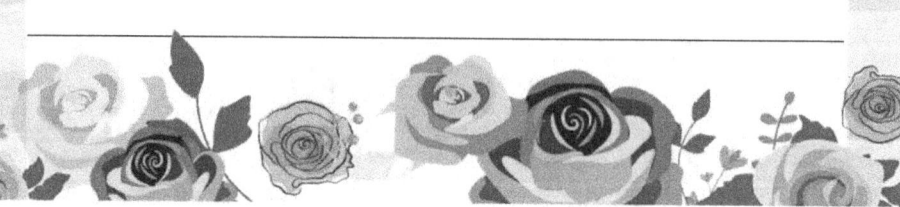

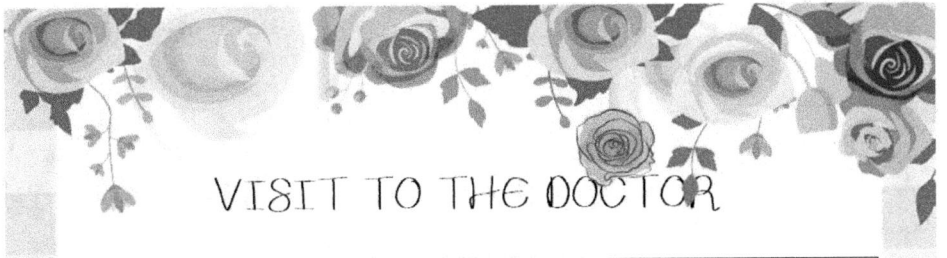

VISIT TO THE DOCTOR

Date	
Doctor	
Hospital or Clinic	
Reason for Visit	
Diasnosis	
Doctor's Comment & Notes	
Follow Up	

Date	
Doctor	
Hospital or Clinic	
Reason for Visit	
Diasnosis	
Doctor,s Comment & Notes	
Follow Up	

Date	
Doctor	
Hospital or Clinic	
Reason for Visit	
Diasnosis	
Doctor's Comment & Notes	
Follow Up	

Date	
Doctor	
Hospital or Clinic	
Reason for Visit	
Diasnosis	
Doctor's Comment & Notes	
Follow Up	

Notes:

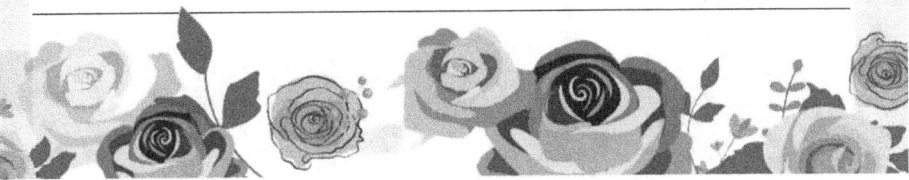

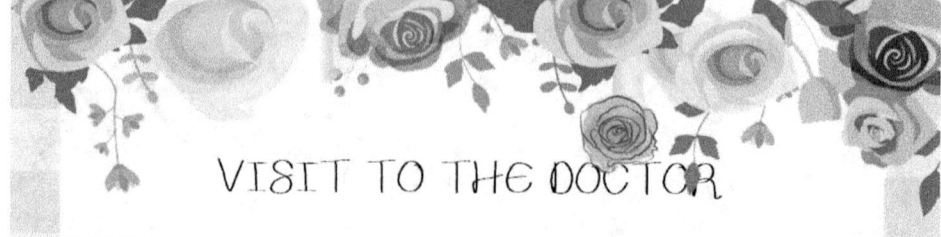

VISIT TO THE DOCTOR

Date	
Doctor	
Hospital or Clinic	
Reason for Visit	
Diasnosis	
Doctor's Comment & Notes	
Follow Up	

Date	
Doctor	
Hospital or Clinic	
Reason for Visit	
Diasnosis	
Doctor,s Comment & Notes	
Follow Up	

Date	
Doctor	
Hospital or Clinic	
Reason for Visit	
Diasnosis	
Doctor's Comment & Notes	
Follow Up	

Date	
Doctor	
Hospital or Clinic	
Reason for Visit	
Diasnosis	
Doctor's Comment & Notes	
Follow Up	

Notes:

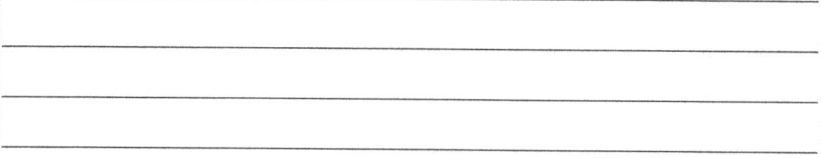

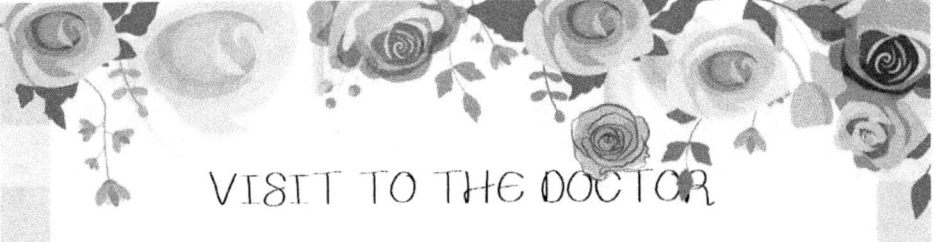

VISIT TO THE DOCTOR

Date	
Doctor	
Hospital or Clinic	
Reason for Visit	
Diasnosis	
Doctor's Comment & Notes	
Follow Up	

Date	
Doctor	
Hospital or Clinic	
Reason for Visit	
Diasnosis	
Doctor,s Comment & Notes	
Follow Up	

Date	
Doctor	
Hospital or Clinic	
Reason for Visit	
Diasnosis	
Doctor's Comment & Notes	
Follow Up	

Date	
Doctor	
Hospital or Clinic	
Reason for Visit	
Diasnosis	
Doctor's Comment & Notes	
Follow Up	

Notes:

_____

_____

_____

_____

_____

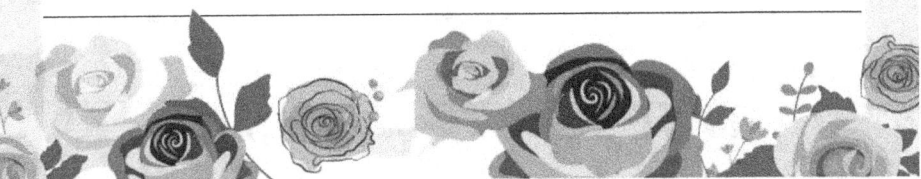

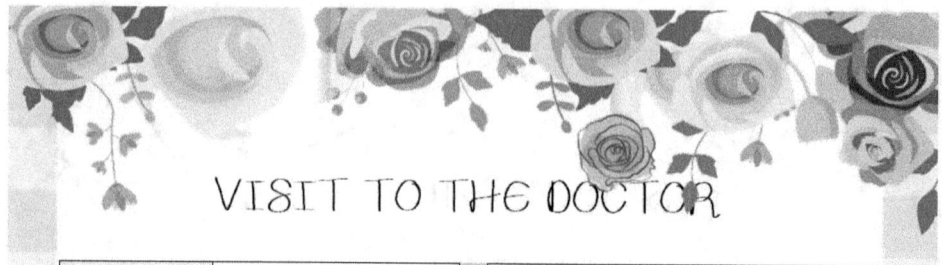

VISIT TO THE DOCTOR

Date	
Doctor	
Hospital or Clinic	
Reason for Visit	
Diasnosis	
Doctor's Comment & Notes	
Follow Up	

Date	
Doctor	
Hospital or Clinic	
Reason for Visit	
Diasnosis	
Doctor,s Comment & Notes	
Follow Up	

Date	
Doctor	
Hospital or Clinic	
Reason for Visit	
Diasnosis	
Doctor's Comment & Notes	
Follow Up	

Date	
Doctor	
Hospital or Clinic	
Reason for Visit	
Diasnosis	
Doctor's Comment & Notes	
Follow Up	

Notes:

_____

_____

_____

_____

_____

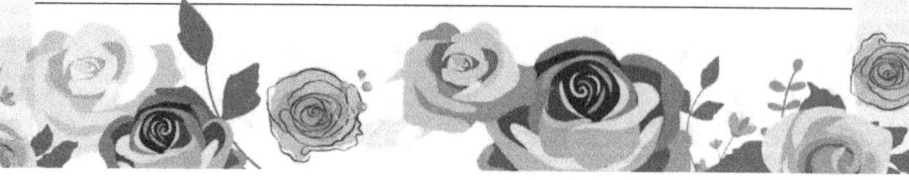

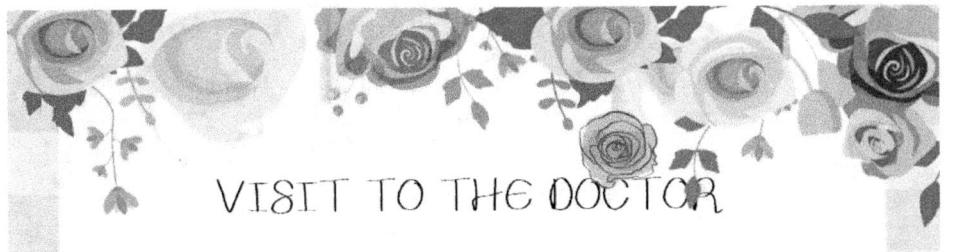

VISIT TO THE DOCTOR

Date	
Doctor	
Hospital or Clinic	
Reason for Visit	
Diasnosis	
Doctor's Comment & Notes	
Follow Up	

Date	
Doctor	
Hospital or Clinic	
Reason for Visit	
Diasnosis	
Doctor,s Comment & Notes	
Follow Up	

Date	
Doctor	
Hospital or Clinic	
Reason for Visit	
Diasnosis	
Doctor's Comment & Notes	
Follow Up	

Date	
Doctor	
Hospital or Clinic	
Reason for Visit	
Diasnosis	
Doctor's Comment & Notes	
Follow Up	

Notes:

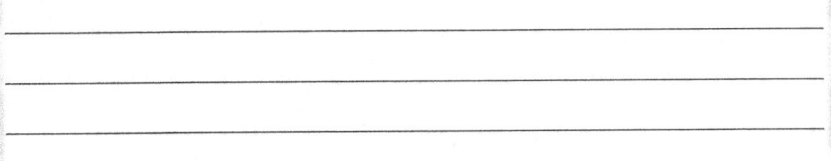
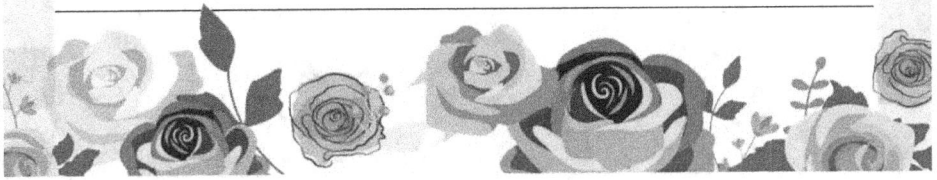

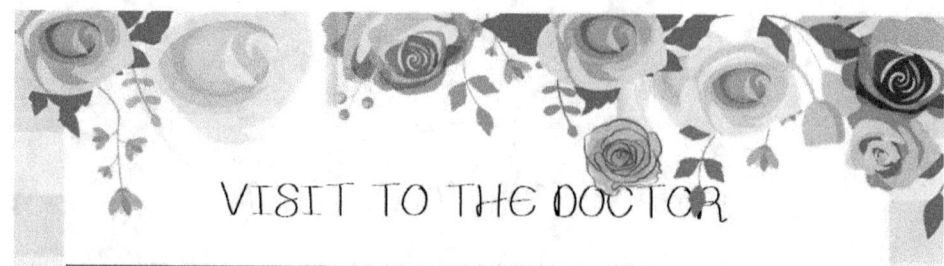

VISIT TO THE DOCTOR

Date	
Doctor	
Hospital or Clinic	
Reason for Visit	
Diasnosis	
Doctor's Comment & Notes	
Follow Up	

Date	
Doctor	
Hospital or Clinic	
Reason for Visit	
Diasnosis	
Doctor,s Comment & Notes	
Follow Up	

Date	
Doctor	
Hospital or Clinic	
Reason for Visit	
Diasnosis	
Doctor's Comment & Notes	
Follow Up	

Date	
Doctor	
Hospital or Clinic	
Reason for Visit	
Diasnosis	
Doctor's Comment & Notes	
Follow Up	

Notes:

_____

_____

_____

_____

_____

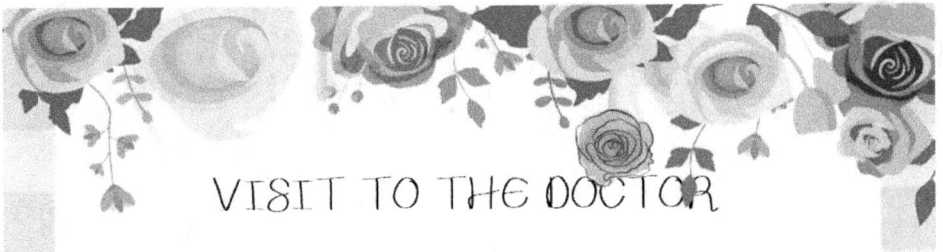

VISIT TO THE DOCTOR

Date	
Doctor	
Hospital or Clinic	
Reason for Visit	
Diasnosis	
Doctor's Comment & Notes	
Follow Up	

Date	
Doctor	
Hospital or Clinic	
Reason for Visit	
Diasnosis	
Doctor,s Comment & Notes	
Follow Up	

Date	
Doctor	
Hospital or Clinic	
Reason for Visit	
Diasnosis	
Doctor's Comment & Notes	
Follow Up	

Date	
Doctor	
Hospital or Clinic	
Reason for Visit	
Diasnosis	
Doctor's Comment & Notes	
Follow Up	

Notes:

_____

_____

_____

_____

_____

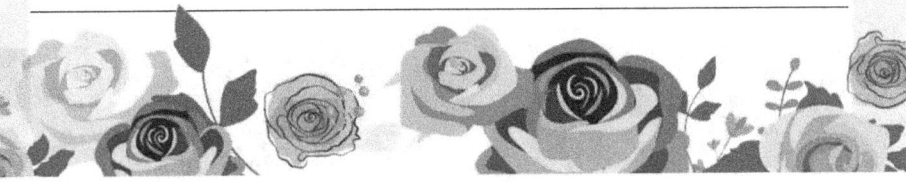

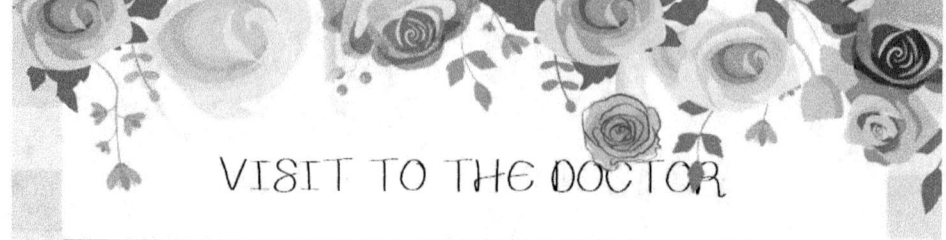

VISIT TO THE DOCTOR

Date	
Doctor	
Hospital or Clinic	
Reason for Visit	
Diasnosis	
Doctor's Comment & Notes	
Follow Up	

Date	
Doctor	
Hospital or Clinic	
Reason for Visit	
Diasnosis	
Doctor,s Comment & Notes	
Follow Up	

Date	
Doctor	
Hospital or Clinic	
Reason for Visit	
Diasnosis	
Doctor's Comment & Notes	
Follow Up	

Date	
Doctor	
Hospital or Clinic	
Reason for Visit	
Diasnosis	
Doctor's Comment & Notes	
Follow Up	

Notes:

_____

_____

_____

_____

_____

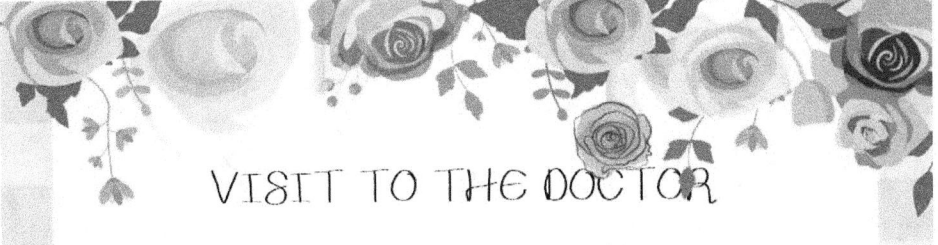

VISIT TO THE DOCTOR

Date			Date	
Doctor			Doctor	
Hospital or Clinic			Hospital or Clinic	
Reason for Visit			Reason for Visit	
Diasnosis			Diasnosis	
Doctor's Comment & Notes			Doctor,s Comment & Notes	
Follow Up			Follow Up	

Date			Date	
Doctor			Doctor	
Hospital or Clinic			Hospital or Clinic	
Reason for Visit			Reason for Visit	
Diasnosis			Diasnosis	
Doctor's Comment & Notes			Doctor's Comment & Notes	
Follow Up			Follow Up	

Notes:

_____

_____

_____

_____

_____

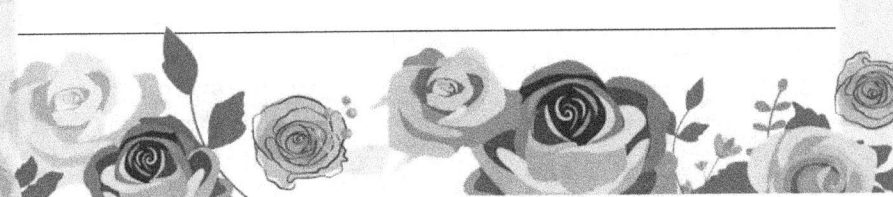

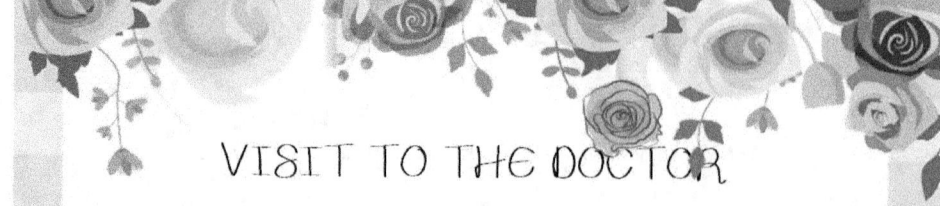

VISIT TO THE DOCTOR

Date	
Doctor	
Hospital or Clinic	
Reason for Visit	
Diasnosis	
Doctor's Comment & Notes	
Follow Up	

Date	
Doctor	
Hospital or Clinic	
Reason for Visit	
Diasnosis	
Doctor,s Comment & Notes	
Follow Up	

Date	
Doctor	
Hospital or Clinic	
Reason for Visit	
Diasnosis	
Doctor's Comment & Notes	
Follow Up	

Date	
Doctor	
Hospital or Clinic	
Reason for Visit	
Diasnosis	
Doctor's Comment & Notes	
Follow Up	

Notes:

_____

_____

_____

_____

_____

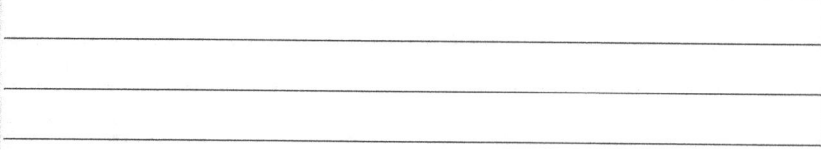
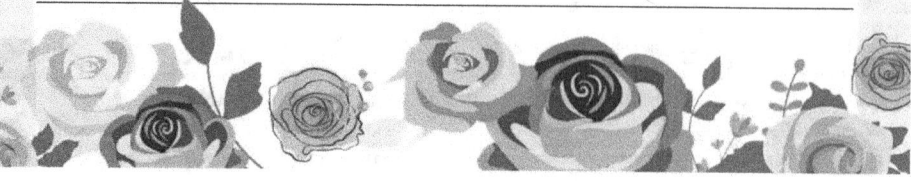

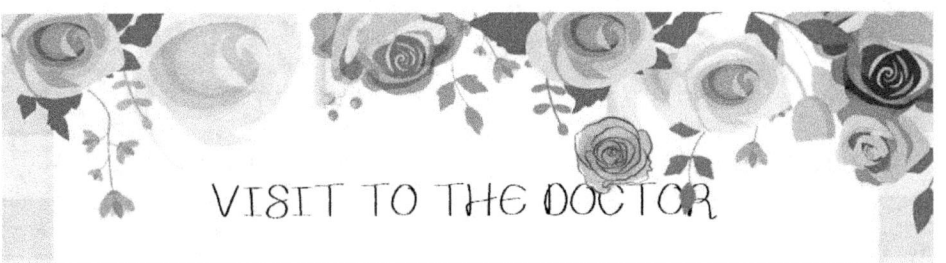

VISIT TO THE DOCTOR

Date	
Doctor	
Hospital or Clinic	
Reason for Visit	
Diasnosis	
Doctor's Comment & Notes	
Follow Up	

Date	
Doctor	
Hospital or Clinic	
Reason for Visit	
Diasnosis	
Doctor,s Comment & Notes	
Follow Up	

Date	
Doctor	
Hospital or Clinic	
Reason for Visit	
Diasnosis	
Doctor's Comment & Notes	
Follow Up	

Date	
Doctor	
Hospital or Clinic	
Reason for Visit	
Diasnosis	
Doctor's Comment & Notes	
Follow Up	

Notes:

_____

_____

_____

_____

_____

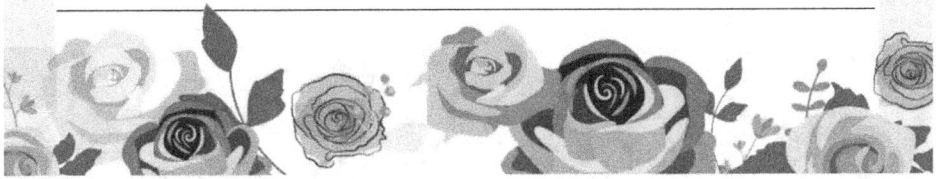

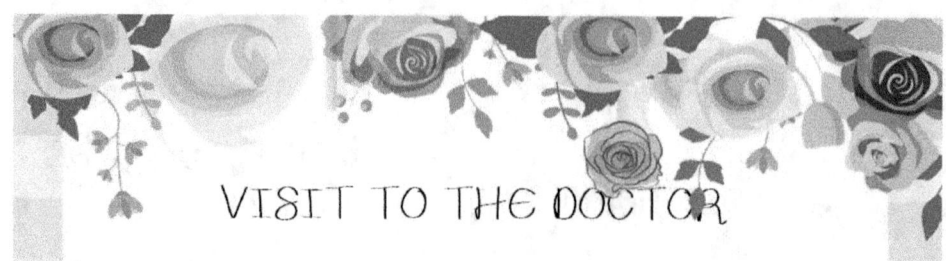

VISIT TO THE DOCTOR

Date	
Doctor	
Hospital or Clinic	
Reason for Visit	
Diasnosis	
Doctor's Comment & Notes	
Follow Up	

Date	
Doctor	
Hospital or Clinic	
Reason for Visit	
Diasnosis	
Doctor,s Comment & Notes	
Follow Up	

Date	
Doctor	
Hospital or Clinic	
Reason for Visit	
Diasnosis	
Doctor's Comment & Notes	
Follow Up	

Date	
Doctor	
Hospital or Clinic	
Reason for Visit	
Diasnosis	
Doctor's Comment & Notes	
Follow Up	

Notes:

_____

_____

_____

_____

_____

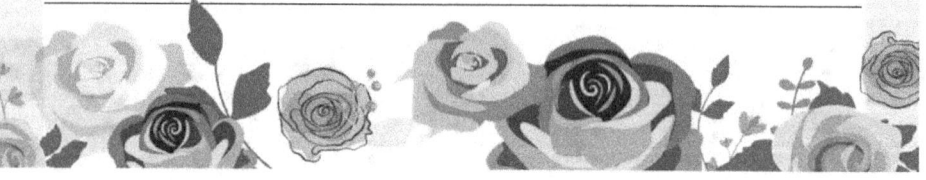

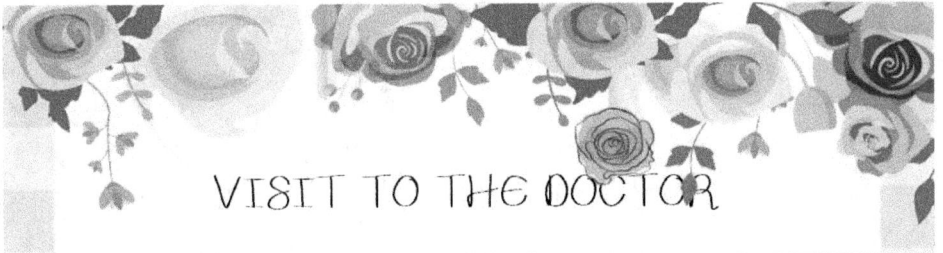

VISIT TO THE DOCTOR

Date	
Doctor	
Hospital or Clinic	
Reason for Visit	
Diasnosis	
Doctor's Comment & Notes	
Follow Up	

Date	
Doctor	
Hospital or Clinic	
Reason for Visit	
Diasnosis	
Doctor,s Comment & Notes	
Follow Up	

Date	
Doctor	
Hospital or Clinic	
Reason for Visit	
Diasnosis	
Doctor's Comment & Notes	
Follow Up	

Date	
Doctor	
Hospital or Clinic	
Reason for Visit	
Diasnosis	
Doctor's Comment & Notes	
Follow Up	

Notes:

_____

_____

_____

_____

_____

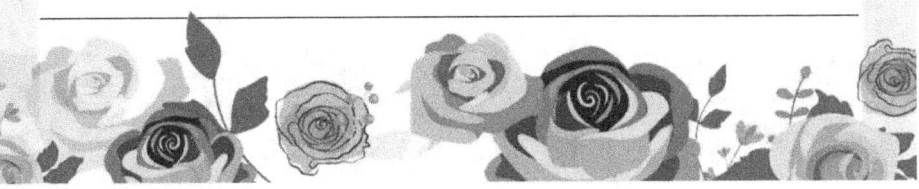

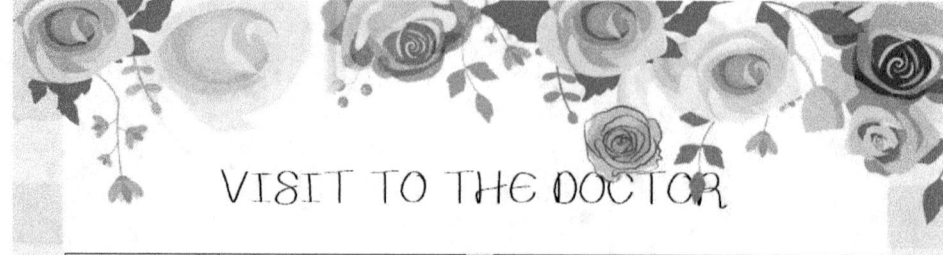

VISIT TO THE DOCTOR

Date			Date	
Doctor			Doctor	
Hospital or Clinic			Hospital or Clinic	
Reason for Visit			Reason for Visit	
Diasnosis			Diasnosis	
Doctor's Comment & Notes			Doctor,s Comment & Notes	
Follow Up			Follow Up	

Date			Date	
Doctor			Doctor	
Hospital or Clinic			Hospital or Clinic	
Reason for Visit			Reason for Visit	
Diasnosis			Diasnosis	
Doctor's Comment & Notes			Doctor's Comment & Notes	
Follow Up			Follow Up	

Notes:

_____

_____

_____

_____

_____

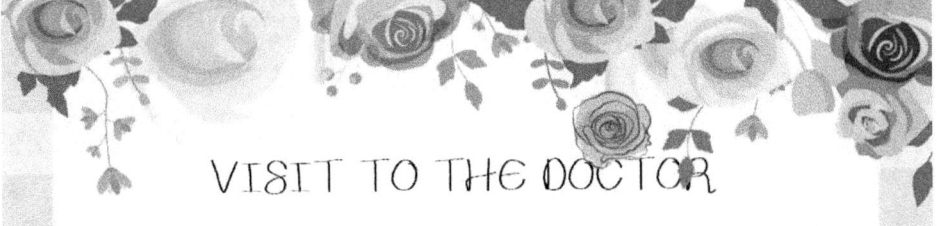

VISIT TO THE DOCTOR

Date	
Doctor	
Hospital or Clinic	
Reason for Visit	
Diasnosis	
Doctor's Comment & Notes	
Follow Up	

Date	
Doctor	
Hospital or Clinic	
Reason for Visit	
Diasnosis	
Doctor,s Comment & Notes	
Follow Up	

Date	
Doctor	
Hospital or Clinic	
Reason for Visit	
Diasnosis	
Doctor's Comment & Notes	
Follow Up	

Date	
Doctor	
Hospital or Clinic	
Reason for Visit	
Diasnosis	
Doctor's Comment & Notes	
Follow Up	

Notes:

_____

_____

_____

_____

_____

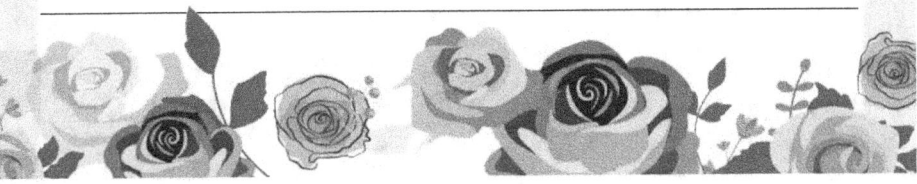

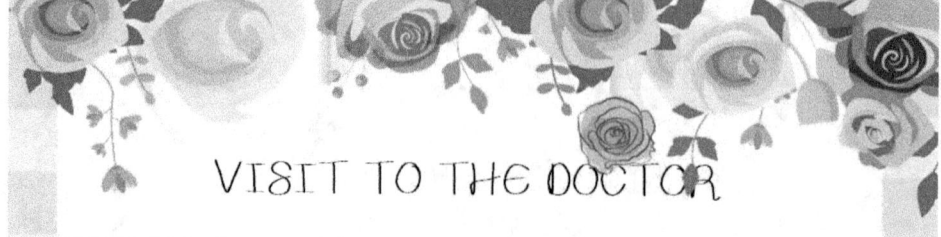

VISIT TO THE DOCTOR

Date	
Doctor	
Hospital or Clinic	
Reason for Visit	
Diasnosis	
Doctor's Comment & Notes	
Follow Up	

Date	
Doctor	
Hospital or Clinic	
Reason for Visit	
Diasnosis	
Doctor,s Comment & Notes	
Follow Up	

Date	
Doctor	
Hospital or Clinic	
Reason for Visit	
Diasnosis	
Doctor's Comment & Notes	
Follow Up	

Date	
Doctor	
Hospital or Clinic	
Reason for Visit	
Diasnosis	
Doctor's Comment & Notes	
Follow Up	

Notes:

_____

_____

_____

_____

_____

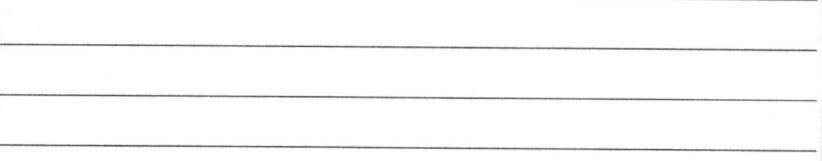

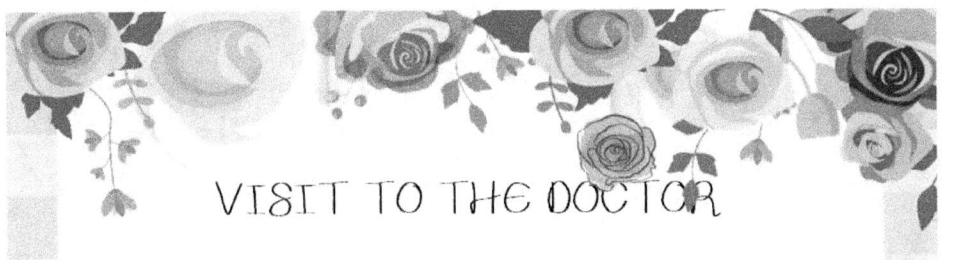

VISIT TO THE DOCTOR

Date	
Doctor	
Hospital or Clinic	
Reason for Visit	
Diasnosis	
Doctor's Comment & Notes	
Follow Up	

Date	
Doctor	
Hospital or Clinic	
Reason for Visit	
Diasnosis	
Doctor,s Comment & Notes	
Follow Up	

Date	
Doctor	
Hospital or Clinic	
Reason for Visit	
Diasnosis	
Doctor's Comment & Notes	
Follow Up	

Date	
Doctor	
Hospital or Clinic	
Reason for Visit	
Diasnosis	
Doctor's Comment & Notes	
Follow Up	

Notes:

_____

_____

_____

_____

_____

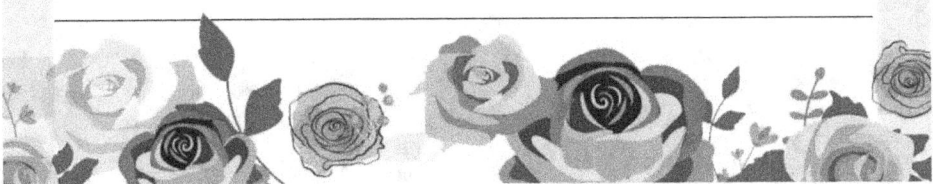

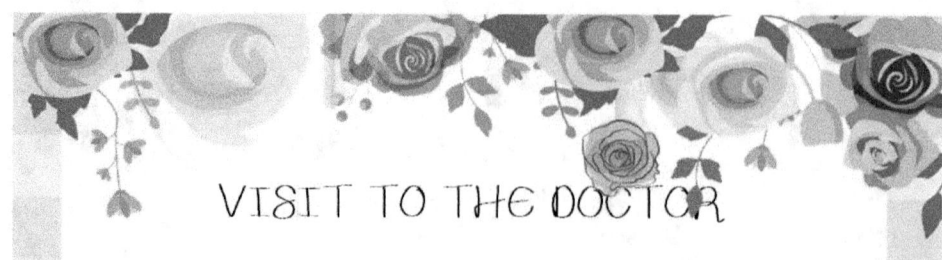

VISIT TO THE DOCTOR

Date			Date	
Doctor			Doctor	
Hospital or Clinic			Hospital or Clinic	
Reason for Visit			Reason for Visit	
Diasnosis			Diasnosis	
Doctor's Comment & Notes			Doctor,s Comment & Notes	
Follow Up			Follow Up	

Date			Date	
Doctor			Doctor	
Hospital or Clinic			Hospital or Clinic	
Reason for Visit			Reason for Visit	
Diasnosis			Diasnosis	
Doctor's Comment & Notes			Doctor's Comment & Notes	
Follow Up			Follow Up	

Notes:

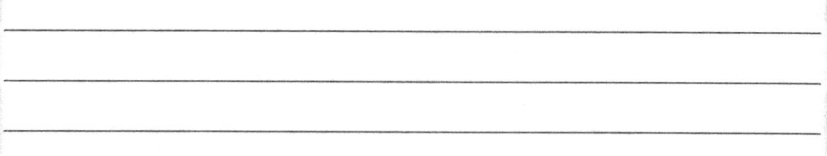

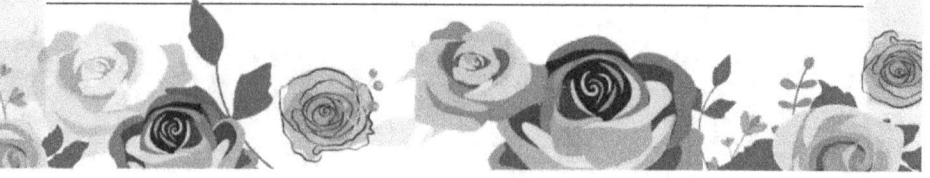

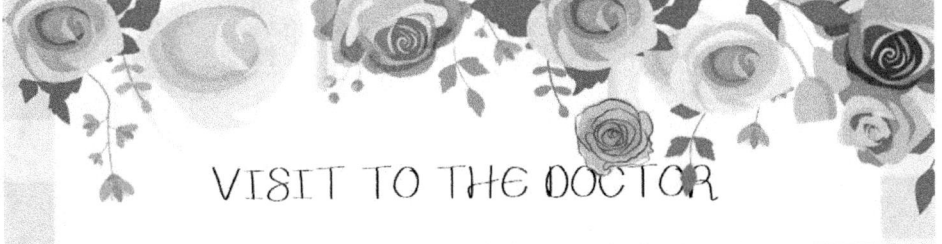

VISIT TO THE DOCTOR

Date	
Doctor	
Hospital or Clinic	
Reason for Visit	
Diasnosis	
Doctor's Comment & Notes	
Follow Up	

Date	
Doctor	
Hospital or Clinic	
Reason for Visit	
Diasnosis	
Doctor,s Comment & Notes	
Follow Up	

Date	
Doctor	
Hospital or Clinic	
Reason for Visit	
Diasnosis	
Doctor's Comment & Notes	
Follow Up	

Date	
Doctor	
Hospital or Clinic	
Reason for Visit	
Diasnosis	
Doctor's Comment & Notes	
Follow Up	

Notes:
_____
_____
_____
_____
_____

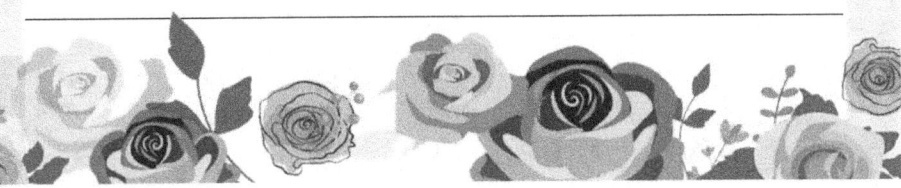

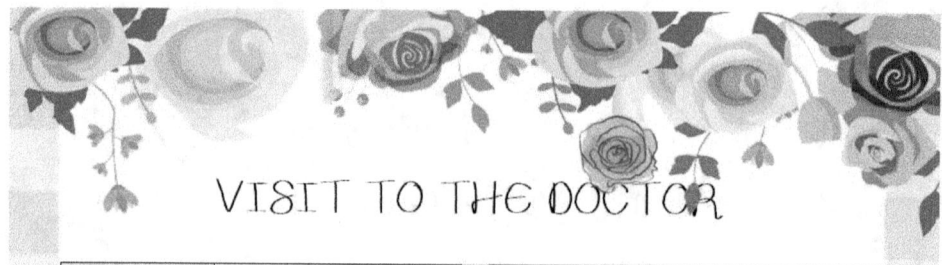

VISIT TO THE DOCTOR

Date	
Doctor	
Hospital or Clinic	
Reason for Visit	
Diasnosis	
Doctor's Comment & Notes	
Follow Up	

Date	
Doctor	
Hospital or Clinic	
Reason for Visit	
Diasnosis	
Doctor,s Comment & Notes	
Follow Up	

Date	
Doctor	
Hospital or Clinic	
Reason for Visit	
Diasnosis	
Doctor's Comment & Notes	
Follow Up	

Date	
Doctor	
Hospital or Clinic	
Reason for Visit	
Diasnosis	
Doctor's Comment & Notes	
Follow Up	

Notes:

_____

_____

_____

_____

_____

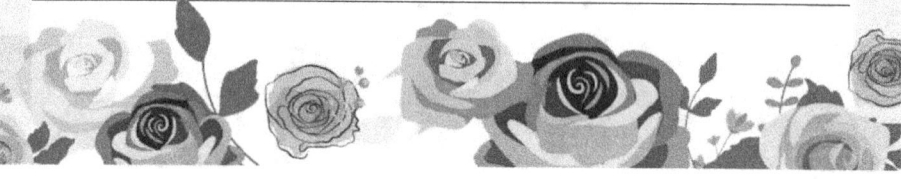

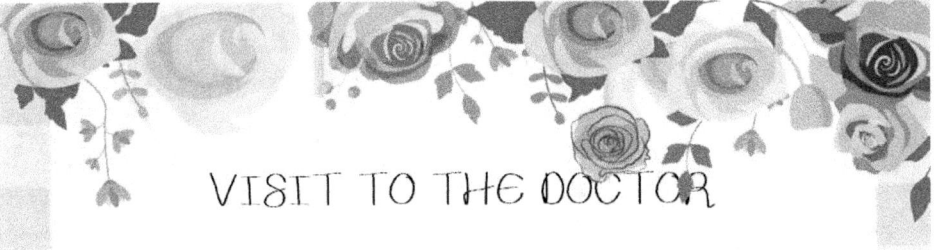

VISIT TO THE DOCTOR

Date	
Doctor	
Hospital or Clinic	
Reason for Visit	
Diasnosis	
Doctor's Comment & Notes	
Follow Up	

Date	
Doctor	
Hospital or Clinic	
Reason for Visit	
Diasnosis	
Doctor,s Comment & Notes	
Follow Up	

Date	
Doctor	
Hospital or Clinic	
Reason for Visit	
Diasnosis	
Doctor's Comment & Notes	
Follow Up	

Date	
Doctor	
Hospital or Clinic	
Reason for Visit	
Diasnosis	
Doctor's Comment & Notes	
Follow Up	

Notes: _____

_____

_____

_____

_____

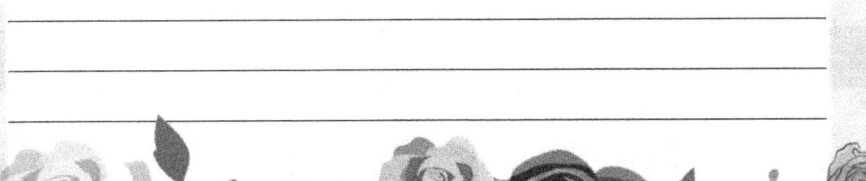

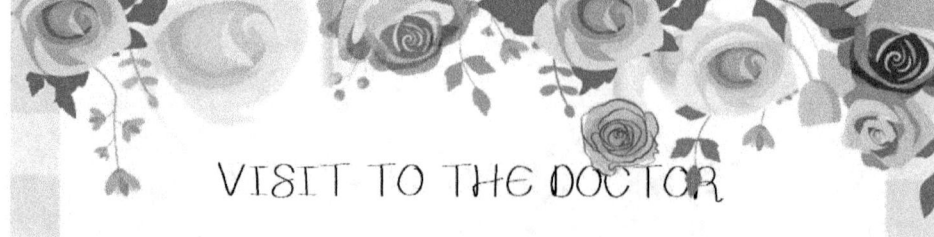

VISIT TO THE DOCTOR

Date	
Doctor	
Hospital or Clinic	
Reason for Visit	
Diasnosis	
Doctor's Comment & Notes	
Follow Up	

Date	
Doctor	
Hospital or Clinic	
Reason for Visit	
Diasnosis	
Doctor,s Comment & Notes	
Follow Up	

Date	
Doctor	
Hospital or Clinic	
Reason for Visit	
Diasnosis	
Doctor's Comment & Notes	
Follow Up	

Date	
Doctor	
Hospital or Clinic	
Reason for Visit	
Diasnosis	
Doctor's Comment & Notes	
Follow Up	

Notes:

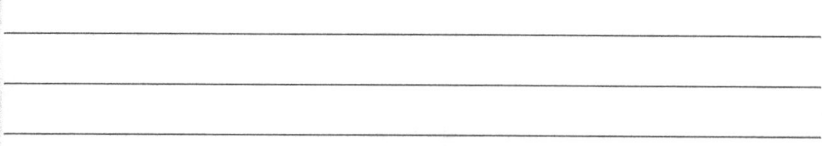

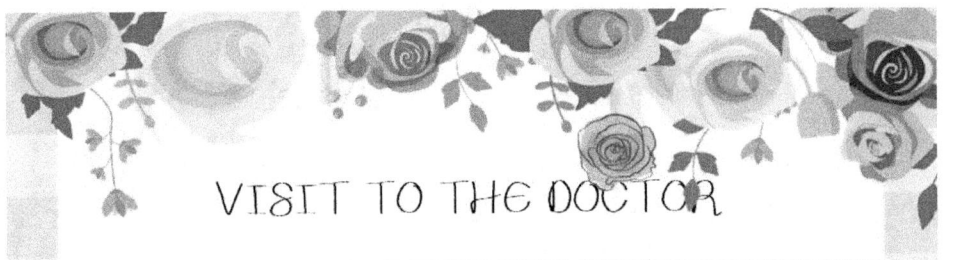

VISIT TO THE DOCTOR

Date	
Doctor	
Hospital or Clinic	
Reason for Visit	
Diasnosis	
Doctor's Comment & Notes	
Follow Up	

Date	
Doctor	
Hospital or Clinic	
Reason for Visit	
Diasnosis	
Doctor,s Comment & Notes	
Follow Up	

Date	
Doctor	
Hospital or Clinic	
Reason for Visit	
Diasnosis	
Doctor's Comment & Notes	
Follow Up	

Date	
Doctor	
Hospital or Clinic	
Reason for Visit	
Diasnosis	
Doctor's Comment & Notes	
Follow Up	

Notes: _____

_____

_____

_____

_____

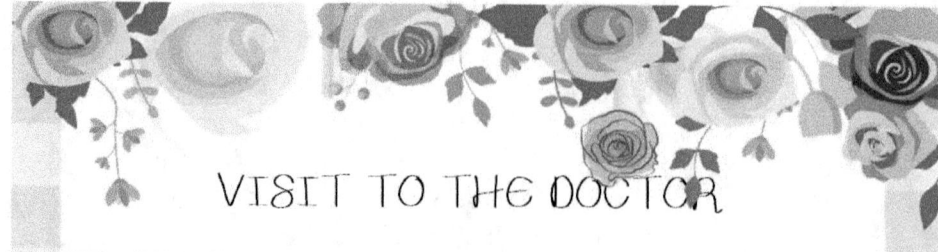

VISIT TO THE DOCTOR

Date	
Doctor	
Hospital or Clinic	
Reason for Visit	
Diasnosis	
Doctor's Comment & Notes	
Follow Up	

Date	
Doctor	
Hospital or Clinic	
Reason for Visit	
Diasnosis	
Doctor,s Comment & Notes	
Follow Up	

Date	
Doctor	
Hospital or Clinic	
Reason for Visit	
Diasnosis	
Doctor's Comment & Notes	
Follow Up	

Date	
Doctor	
Hospital or Clinic	
Reason for Visit	
Diasnosis	
Doctor's Comment & Notes	
Follow Up	

Notes:

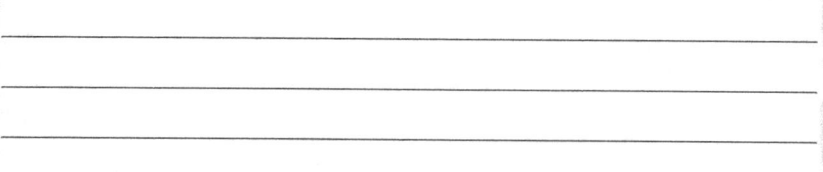

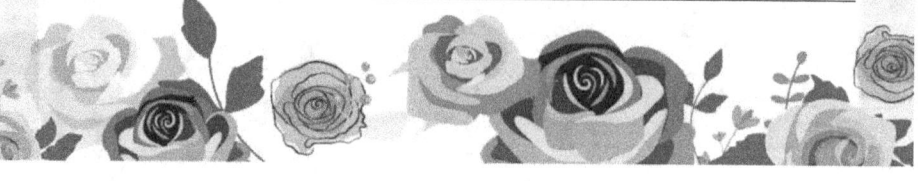

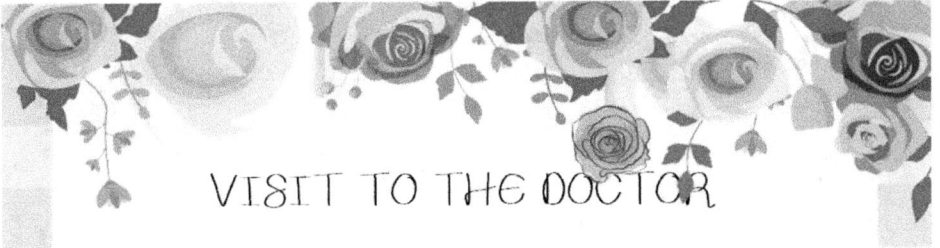

VISIT TO THE DOCTOR

Date	
Doctor	
Hospital or Clinic	
Reason for Visit	
Diasnosis	
Doctor's Comment & Notes	
Follow Up	

Date	
Doctor	
Hospital or Clinic	
Reason for Visit	
Diasnosis	
Doctor,s Comment & Notes	
Follow Up	

Date	
Doctor	
Hospital or Clinic	
Reason for Visit	
Diasnosis	
Doctor's Comment & Notes	
Follow Up	

Date	
Doctor	
Hospital or Clinic	
Reason for Visit	
Diasnosis	
Doctor's Comment & Notes	
Follow Up	

Notes: _____

_____

_____

_____

_____

_____

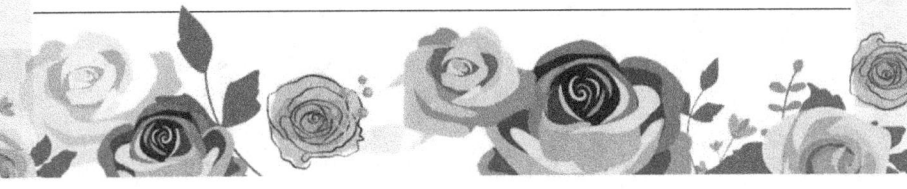

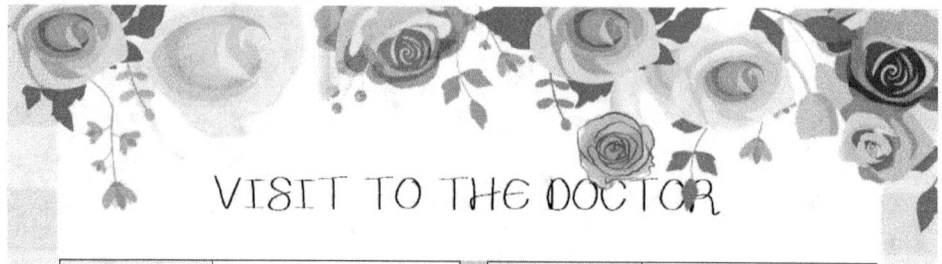

VISIT TO THE DOCTOR

Date	
Doctor	
Hospital or Clinic	
Reason for Visit	
Diasnosis	
Doctor's Comment & Notes	
Follow Up	

Date	
Doctor	
Hospital or Clinic	
Reason for Visit	
Diasnosis	
Doctor,s Comment & Notes	
Follow Up	

Date	
Doctor	
Hospital or Clinic	
Reason for Visit	
Diasnosis	
Doctor's Comment & Notes	
Follow Up	

Date	
Doctor	
Hospital or Clinic	
Reason for Visit	
Diasnosis	
Doctor's Comment & Notes	
Follow Up	

Notes:

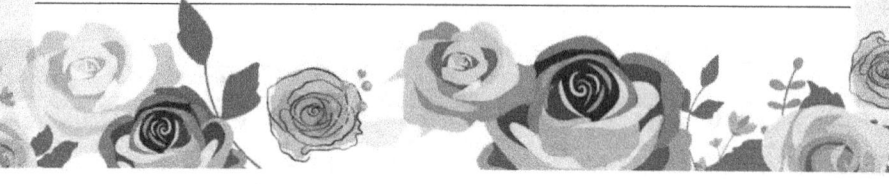

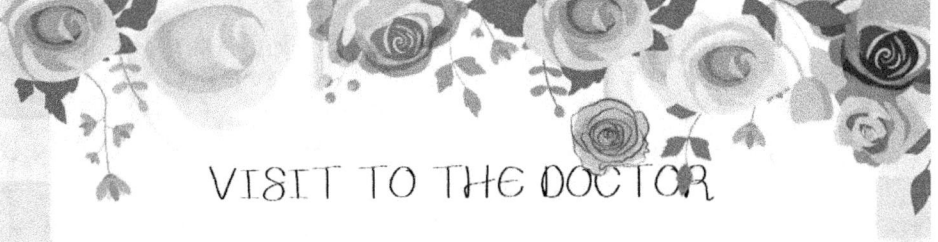

VISIT TO THE DOCTOR

Date		Date	
Doctor		Doctor	
Hospital or Clinic		Hospital or Clinic	
Reason for Visit		Reason for Visit	
Diasnosis		Diasnosis	
Doctor's Comment & Notes		Doctor,s Comment & Notes	
Follow Up		Follow Up	

Date		Date	
Doctor		Doctor	
Hospital or Clinic		Hospital or Clinic	
Reason for Visit		Reason for Visit	
Diasnosis		Diasnosis	
Doctor's Comment & Notes		Doctor's Comment & Notes	
Follow Up		Follow Up	

Notes: _____

_____

_____

_____

_____

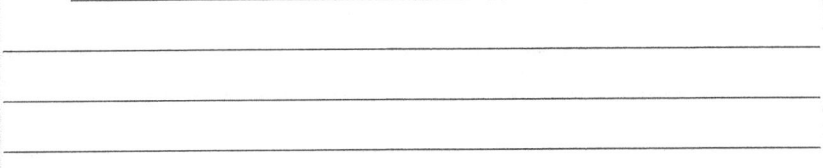
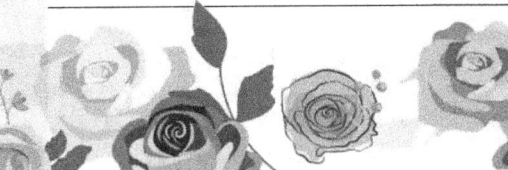
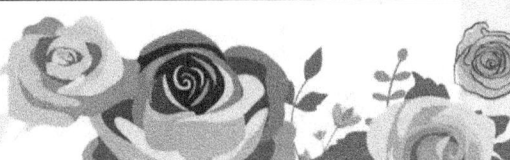

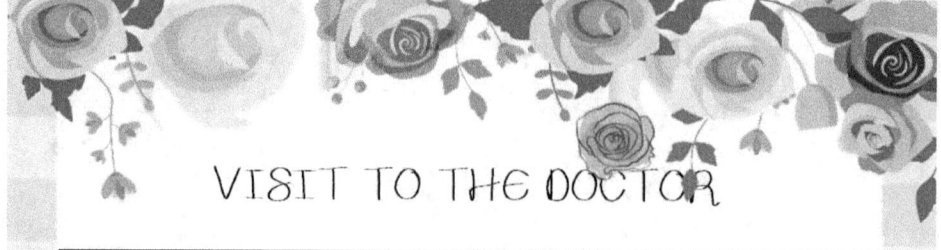

VISIT TO THE DOCTOR

Date			Date	
Doctor			Doctor	
Hospital or Clinic			Hospital or Clinic	
Reason for Visit			Reason for Visit	
Diasnosis			Diasnosis	
Doctor's Comment & Notes			Doctor,s Comment & Notes	
Follow Up			Follow Up	

Date			Date	
Doctor			Doctor	
Hospital or Clinic			Hospital or Clinic	
Reason for Visit			Reason for Visit	
Diasnosis			Diasnosis	
Doctor's Comment & Notes			Doctor's Comment & Notes	
Follow Up			Follow Up	

Notes:
_____
_____
_____
_____
_____

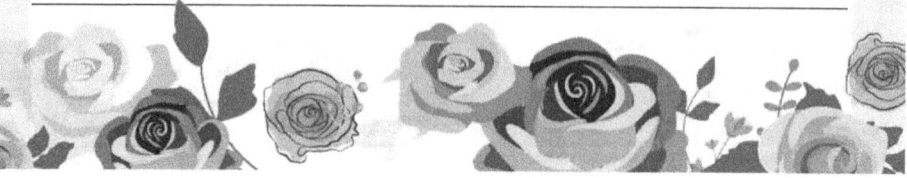

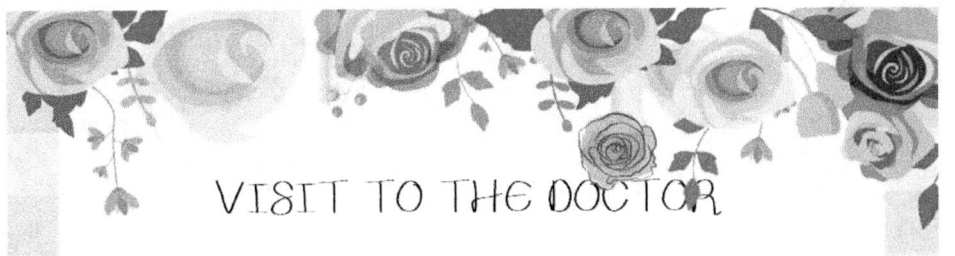

VISIT TO THE DOCTOR

Date	
Doctor	
Hospital or Clinic	
Reason for Visit	
Diasnosis	
Doctor's Comment & Notes	
Follow Up	

Date	
Doctor	
Hospital or Clinic	
Reason for Visit	
Diasnosis	
Doctor,s Comment & Notes	
Follow Up	

Date	
Doctor	
Hospital or Clinic	
Reason for Visit	
Diasnosis	
Doctor's Comment & Notes	
Follow Up	

Date	
Doctor	
Hospital or Clinic	
Reason for Visit	
Diasnosis	
Doctor's Comment & Notes	
Follow Up	

Notes:
_____
_____
_____
_____
_____
_____

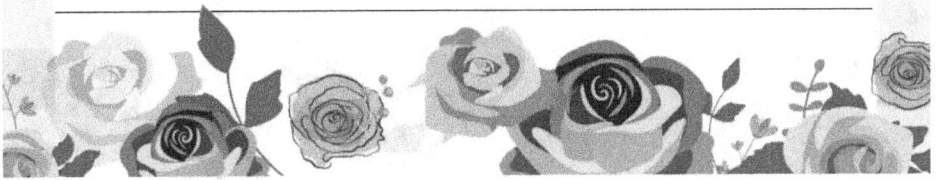

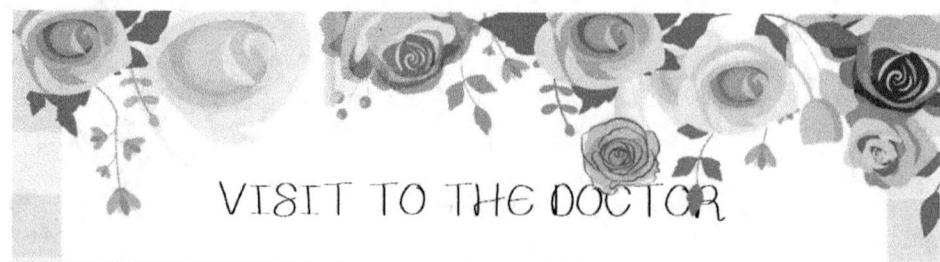

VISIT TO THE DOCTOR

Date	
Doctor	
Hospital or Clinic	
Reason for Visit	
Diasnosis	
Doctor's Comment & Notes	
Follow Up	

Date	
Doctor	
Hospital or Clinic	
Reason for Visit	
Diasnosis	
Doctor,s Comment & Notes	
Follow Up	

Date	
Doctor	
Hospital or Clinic	
Reason for Visit	
Diasnosis	
Doctor's Comment & Notes	
Follow Up	

Date	
Doctor	
Hospital or Clinic	
Reason for Visit	
Diasnosis	
Doctor's Comment & Notes	
Follow Up	

Notes:

_____

_____

_____

_____

_____

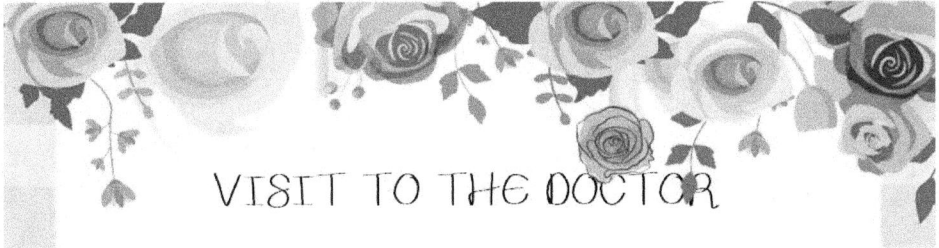

VISIT TO THE DOCTOR

Date	
Doctor	
Hospital or Clinic	
Reason for Visit	
Diasnosis	
Doctor's Comment & Notes	
Follow Up	

Date	
Doctor	
Hospital or Clinic	
Reason for Visit	
Diasnosis	
Doctor,s Comment & Notes	
Follow Up	

Date	
Doctor	
Hospital or Clinic	
Reason for Visit	
Diasnosis	
Doctor's Comment & Notes	
Follow Up	

Date	
Doctor	
Hospital or Clinic	
Reason for Visit	
Diasnosis	
Doctor's Comment & Notes	
Follow Up	

Notes:

_____

_____

_____

_____

_____

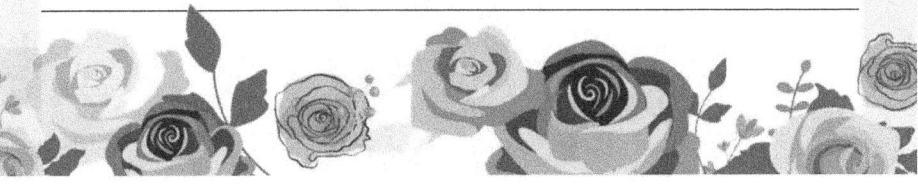

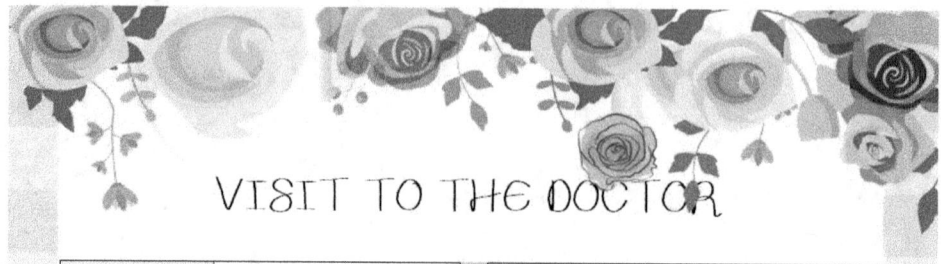

VISIT TO THE DOCTOR

Date	
Doctor	
Hospital or Clinic	
Reason for Visit	
Diasnosis	
Doctor's Comment & Notes	
Follow Up	

Date	
Doctor	
Hospital or Clinic	
Reason for Visit	
Diasnosis	
Doctor,s Comment & Notes	
Follow Up	

Date	
Doctor	
Hospital or Clinic	
Reason for Visit	
Diasnosis	
Doctor's Comment & Notes	
Follow Up	

Date	
Doctor	
Hospital or Clinic	
Reason for Visit	
Diasnosis	
Doctor's Comment & Notes	
Follow Up	

Notes:

_____

_____

_____

_____

_____

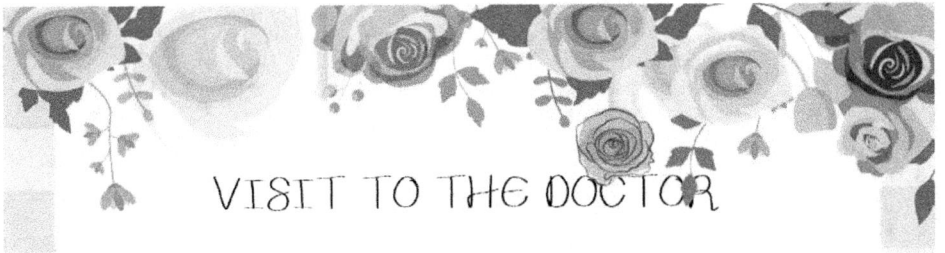

VISIT TO THE DOCTOR

Date			Date	
Doctor			Doctor	
Hospital or Clinic			Hospital or Clinic	
Reason for Visit			Reason for Visit	
Diasnosis			Diasnosis	
Doctor's Comment & Notes			Doctor,s Comment & Notes	
Follow Up			Follow Up	

Date			Date	
Doctor			Doctor	
Hospital or Clinic			Hospital or Clinic	
Reason for Visit			Reason for Visit	
Diasnosis			Diasnosis	
Doctor's Comment & Notes			Doctor's Comment & Notes	
Follow Up			Follow Up	

Notes: _____

_____

_____

_____

_____

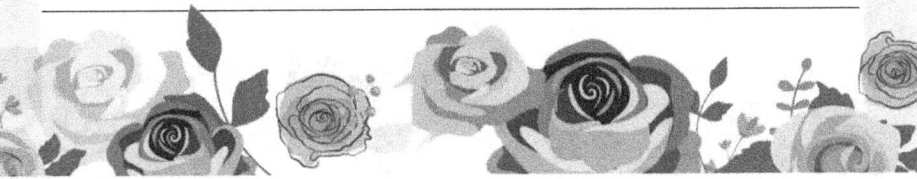

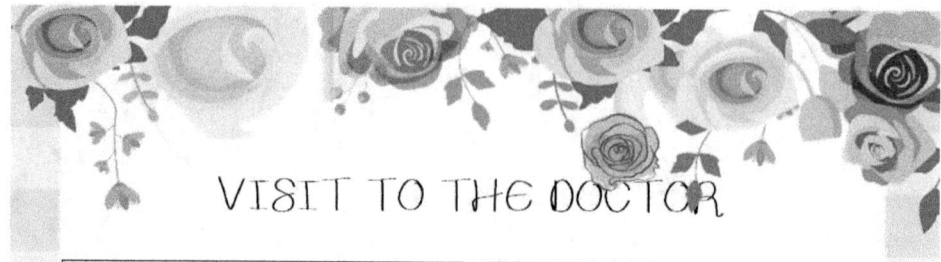

VISIT TO THE DOCTOR

Date	
Doctor	
Hospital or Clinic	
Reason for Visit	
Diasnosis	
Doctor's Comment & Notes	
Follow Up	

Date	
Doctor	
Hospital or Clinic	
Reason for Visit	
Diasnosis	
Doctor,s Comment & Notes	
Follow Up	

Date	
Doctor	
Hospital or Clinic	
Reason for Visit	
Diasnosis	
Doctor's Comment & Notes	
Follow Up	

Date	
Doctor	
Hospital or Clinic	
Reason for Visit	
Diasnosis	
Doctor's Comment & Notes	
Follow Up	

Notes:

_____

_____

_____

_____

_____

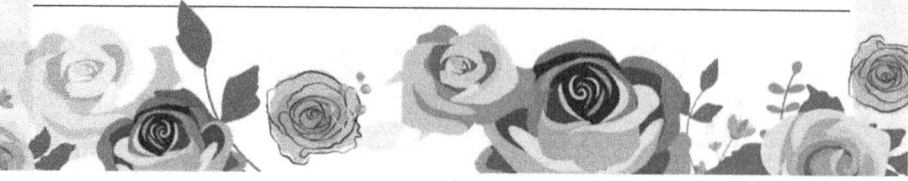

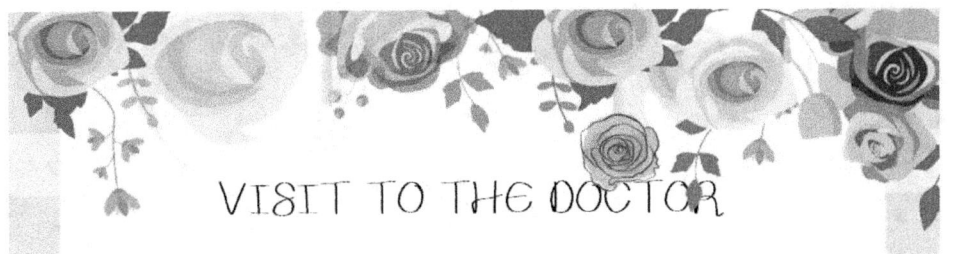

VISIT TO THE DOCTOR

Date	
Doctor	
Hospital or Clinic	
Reason for Visit	
Diasnosis	
Doctor's Comment & Notes	
Follow Up	

Date	
Doctor	
Hospital or Clinic	
Reason for Visit	
Diasnosis	
Doctor,s Comment & Notes	
Follow Up	

Date	
Doctor	
Hospital or Clinic	
Reason for Visit	
Diasnosis	
Doctor's Comment & Notes	
Follow Up	

Date	
Doctor	
Hospital or Clinic	
Reason for Visit	
Diasnosis	
Doctor's Comment & Notes	
Follow Up	

Notes: _____

_____

_____

_____

_____

_____

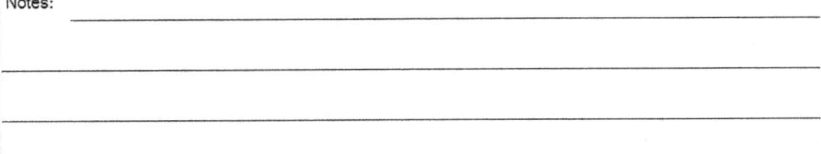

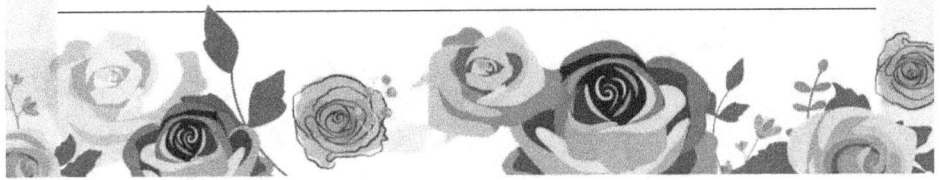

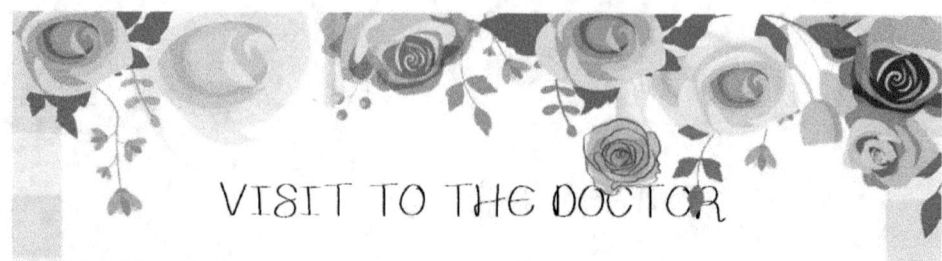

VISIT TO THE DOCTOR

Date	
Doctor	
Hospital or Clinic	
Reason for Visit	
Diasnosis	
Doctor's Comment & Notes	
Follow Up	

Date	
Doctor	
Hospital or Clinic	
Reason for Visit	
Diasnosis	
Doctor,s Comment & Notes	
Follow Up	

Date	
Doctor	
Hospital or Clinic	
Reason for Visit	
Diasnosis	
Doctor's Comment & Notes	
Follow Up	

Date	
Doctor	
Hospital or Clinic	
Reason for Visit	
Diasnosis	
Doctor's Comment & Notes	
Follow Up	

Notes:

_____

_____

_____

_____

_____

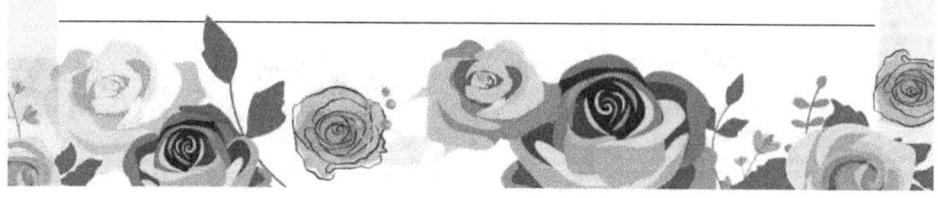

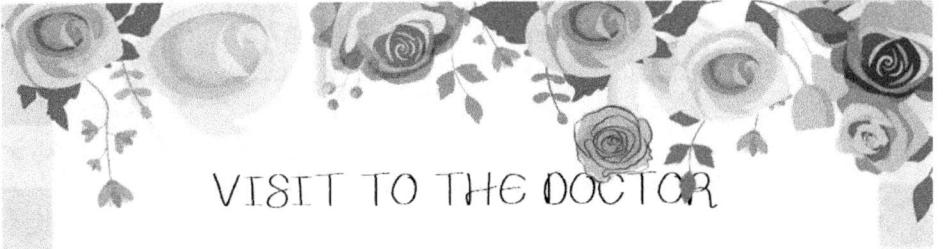

VISIT TO THE DOCTOR

Date	
Doctor	
Hospital or Clinic	
Reason for Visit	
Diasnosis	
Doctor's Comment & Notes	
Follow Up	

Date	
Doctor	
Hospital or Clinic	
Reason for Visit	
Diasnosis	
Doctor,s Comment & Notes	
Follow Up	

Date	
Doctor	
Hospital or Clinic	
Reason for Visit	
Diasnosis	
Doctor's Comment & Notes	
Follow Up	

Date	
Doctor	
Hospital or Clinic	
Reason for Visit	
Diasnosis	
Doctor's Comment & Notes	
Follow Up	

Notes: _____

_____

_____

_____

_____

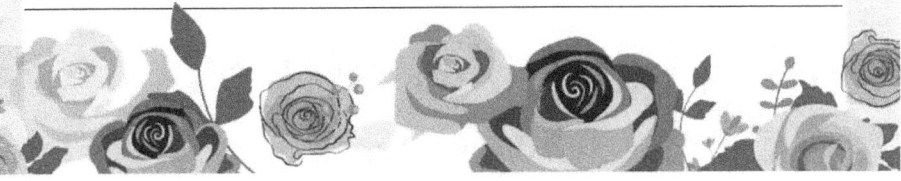

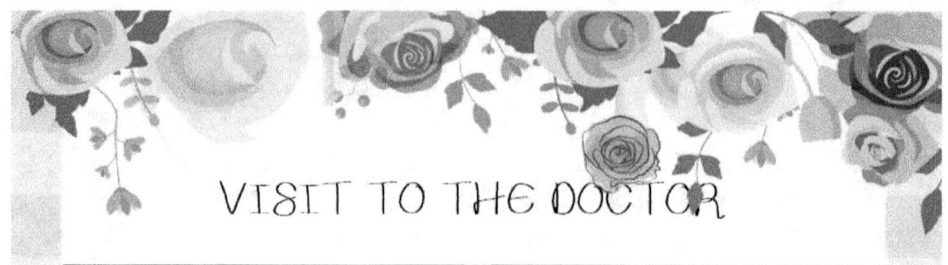

VISIT TO THE DOCTOR

Date	
Doctor	
Hospital or Clinic	
Reason for Visit	
Diasnosis	
Doctor's Comment & Notes	
Follow Up	

Date	
Doctor	
Hospital or Clinic	
Reason for Visit	
Diasnosis	
Doctor,s Comment & Notes	
Follow Up	

Date	
Doctor	
Hospital or Clinic	
Reason for Visit	
Diasnosis	
Doctor's Comment & Notes	
Follow Up	

Date	
Doctor	
Hospital or Clinic	
Reason for Visit	
Diasnosis	
Doctor's Comment & Notes	
Follow Up	

Notes:

_____

_____

_____

_____

_____

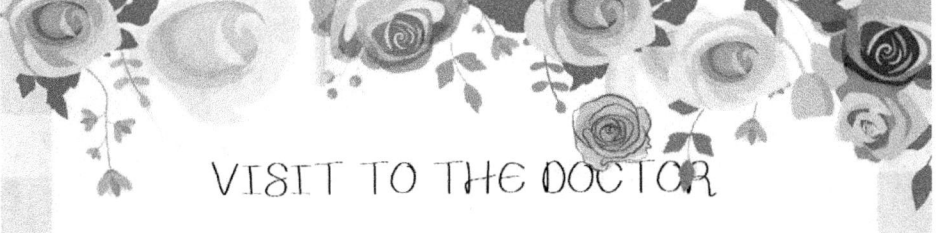

VISIT TO THE DOCTOR

Date	
Doctor	
Hospital or Clinic	
Reason for Visit	
Diasnosis	
Doctor's Comment & Notes	
Follow Up	

Date	
Doctor	
Hospital or Clinic	
Reason for Visit	
Diasnosis	
Doctor,s Comment & Notes	
Follow Up	

Date	
Doctor	
Hospital or Clinic	
Reason for Visit	
Diasnosis	
Doctor's Comment & Notes	
Follow Up	

Date	
Doctor	
Hospital or Clinic	
Reason for Visit	
Diasnosis	
Doctor's Comment & Notes	
Follow Up	

Notes:

_____

_____

_____

_____

_____

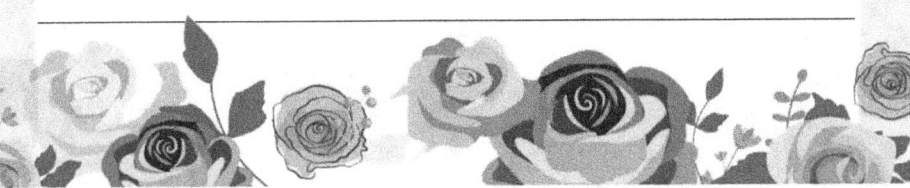

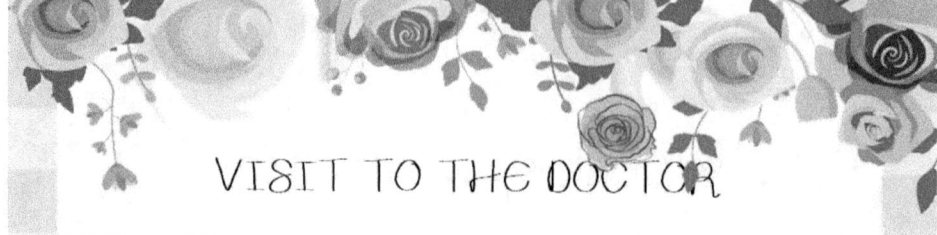

VISIT TO THE DOCTOR

Date	
Doctor	
Hospital or Clinic	
Reason for Visit	
Diasnosis	
Doctor's Comment & Notes	
Follow Up	

Date	
Doctor	
Hospital or Clinic	
Reason for Visit	
Diasnosis	
Doctor,s Comment & Notes	
Follow Up	

Date	
Doctor	
Hospital or Clinic	
Reason for Visit	
Diasnosis	
Doctor's Comment & Notes	
Follow Up	

Date	
Doctor	
Hospital or Clinic	
Reason for Visit	
Diasnosis	
Doctor's Comment & Notes	
Follow Up	

Notes:

_____

_____

_____

_____

_____

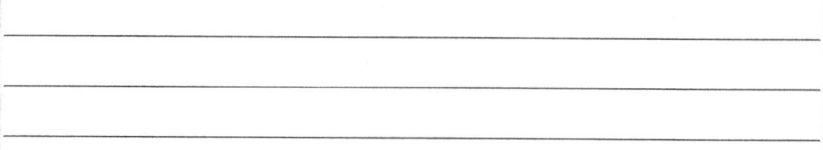

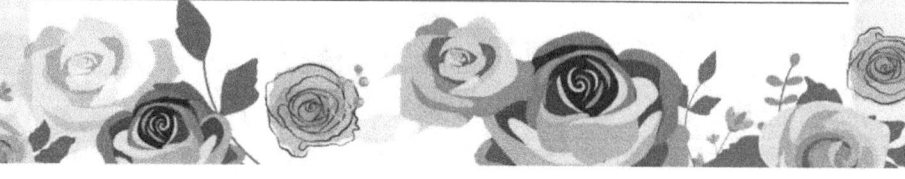

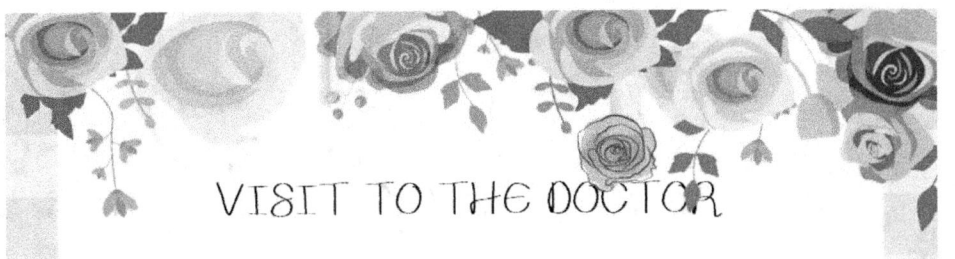

VISIT TO THE DOCTOR

Date	
Doctor	
Hospital or Clinic	
Reason for Visit	
Diasnosis	
Doctor's Comment & Notes	
Follow Up	

Date	
Doctor	
Hospital or Clinic	
Reason for Visit	
Diasnosis	
Doctor,s Comment & Notes	
Follow Up	

Date	
Doctor	
Hospital or Clinic	
Reason for Visit	
Diasnosis	
Doctor's Comment & Notes	
Follow Up	

Date	
Doctor	
Hospital or Clinic	
Reason for Visit	
Diasnosis	
Doctor's Comment & Notes	
Follow Up	

Notes:

_____

_____

_____

_____

_____

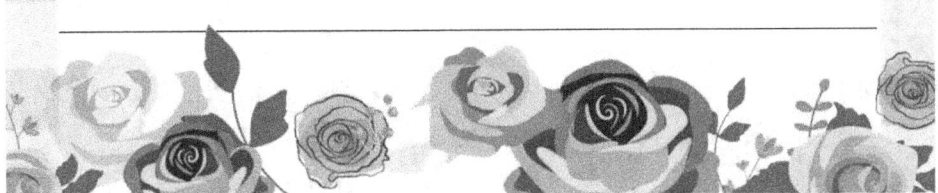

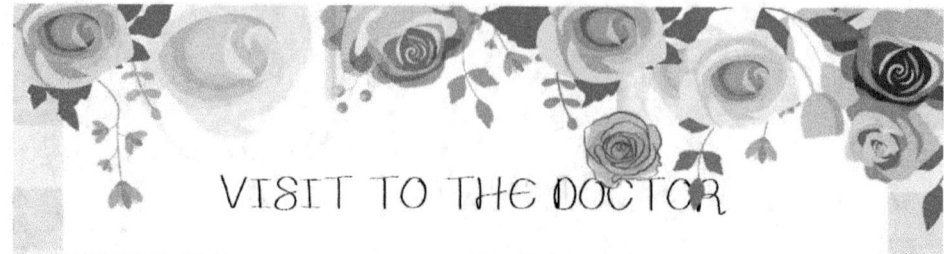

VISIT TO THE DOCTOR

Date	
Doctor	
Hospital or Clinic	
Reason for Visit	
Diasnosis	
Doctor's Comment & Notes	
Follow Up	

Date	
Doctor	
Hospital or Clinic	
Reason for Visit	
Diasnosis	
Doctor,s Comment & Notes	
Follow Up	

Date	
Doctor	
Hospital or Clinic	
Reason for Visit	
Diasnosis	
Doctor's Comment & Notes	
Follow Up	

Date	
Doctor	
Hospital or Clinic	
Reason for Visit	
Diasnosis	
Doctor's Comment & Notes	
Follow Up	

Notes:

_____

_____

_____

_____

_____

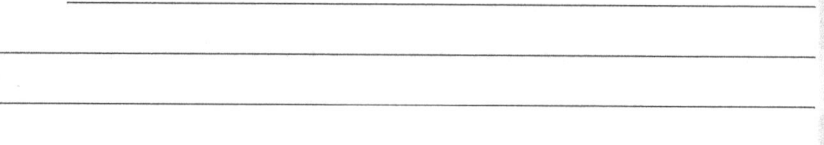

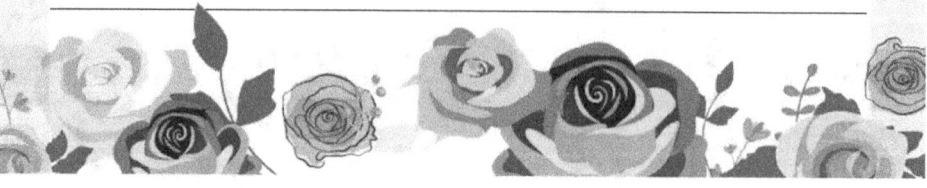

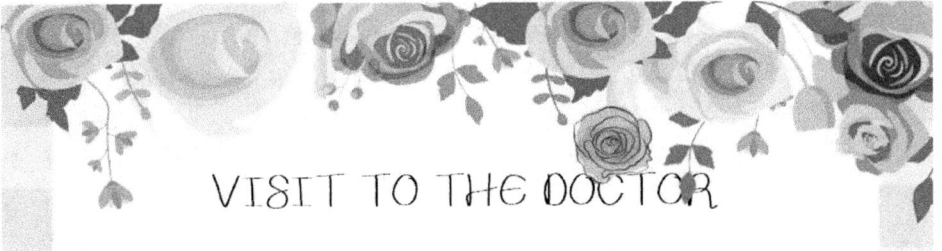

VISIT TO THE DOCTOR

Date	
Doctor	
Hospital or Clinic	
Reason for Visit	
Diasnosis	
Doctor's Comment & Notes	
Follow Up	

Date	
Doctor	
Hospital or Clinic	
Reason for Visit	
Diasnosis	
Doctor,s Comment & Notes	
Follow Up	

Date	
Doctor	
Hospital or Clinic	
Reason for Visit	
Diasnosis	
Doctor's Comment & Notes	
Follow Up	

Date	
Doctor	
Hospital or Clinic	
Reason for Visit	
Diasnosis	
Doctor's Comment & Notes	
Follow Up	

Notes:

_____

_____

_____

_____

_____

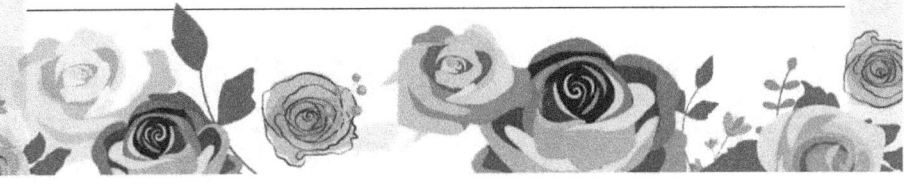

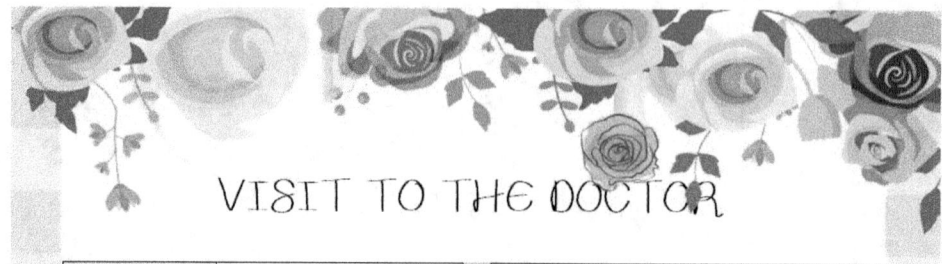

VISIT TO THE DOCTOR

Date	
Doctor	
Hospital or Clinic	
Reason for Visit	
Diasnosis	
Doctor's Comment & Notes	
Follow Up	

Date	
Doctor	
Hospital or Clinic	
Reason for Visit	
Diasnosis	
Doctor,s Comment & Notes	
Follow Up	

Date	
Doctor	
Hospital or Clinic	
Reason for Visit	
Diasnosis	
Doctor's Comment & Notes	
Follow Up	

Date	
Doctor	
Hospital or Clinic	
Reason for Visit	
Diasnosis	
Doctor's Comment & Notes	
Follow Up	

Notes:

_____

_____

_____

_____

_____

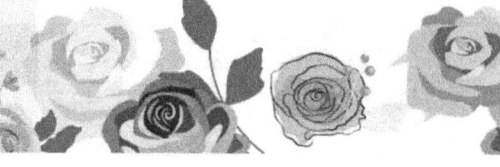
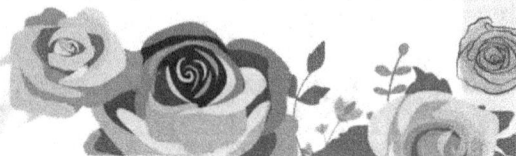

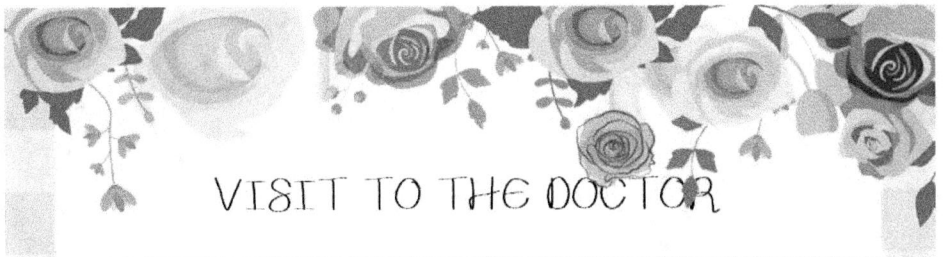

VISIT TO THE DOCTOR

Date			Date	
Doctor			Doctor	
Hospital or Clinic			Hospital or Clinic	
Reason for Visit			Reason for Visit	
Diasnosis			Diasnosis	
Doctor's Comment & Notes			Doctor,s Comment & Notes	
Follow Up			Follow Up	

Date			Date	
Doctor			Doctor	
Hospital or Clinic			Hospital or Clinic	
Reason for Visit			Reason for Visit	
Diasnosis			Diasnosis	
Doctor's Comment & Notes			Doctor's Comment & Notes	
Follow Up			Follow Up	

Notes:

_____

_____

_____

_____

_____

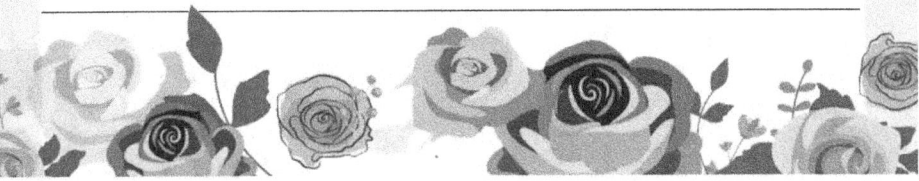

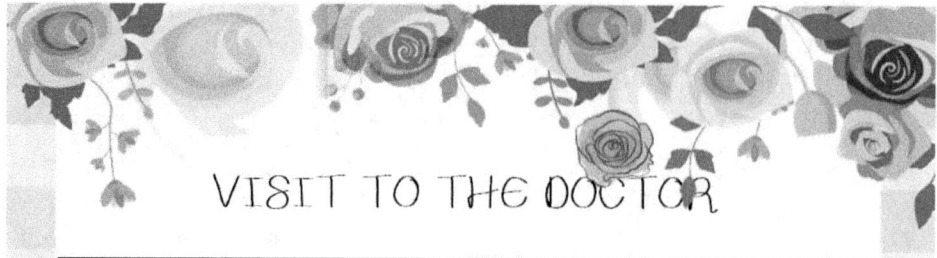

VISIT TO THE DOCTOR

Date	
Doctor	
Hospital or Clinic	
Reason for Visit	
Diasnosis	
Doctor's Comment & Notes	
Follow Up	

Date	
Doctor	
Hospital or Clinic	
Reason for Visit	
Diasnosis	
Doctor,s Comment & Notes	
Follow Up	

Date	
Doctor	
Hospital or Clinic	
Reason for Visit	
Diasnosis	
Doctor's Comment & Notes	
Follow Up	

Date	
Doctor	
Hospital or Clinic	
Reason for Visit	
Diasnosis	
Doctor's Comment & Notes	
Follow Up	

Notes:
_____
_____
_____
_____
_____

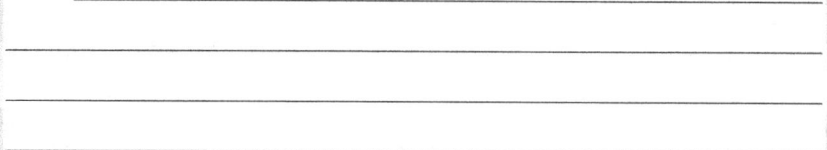

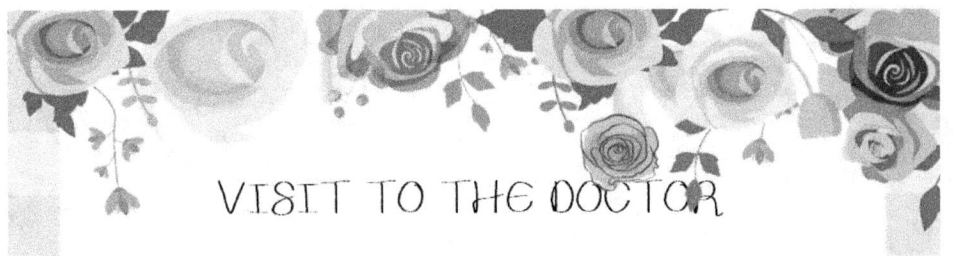

VISIT TO THE DOCTOR

Date			Date	
Doctor			Doctor	
Hospital or Clinic			Hospital or Clinic	
Reason for Visit			Reason for Visit	
Diasnosis			Diasnosis	
Doctor's Comment & Notes			Doctor,s Comment & Notes	
Follow Up			Follow Up	

Date			Date	
Doctor			Doctor	
Hospital or Clinic			Hospital or Clinic	
Reason for Visit			Reason for Visit	
Diasnosis			Diasnosis	
Doctor's Comment & Notes			Doctor's Comment & Notes	
Follow Up			Follow Up	

Notes: _____

_____

_____

_____

_____

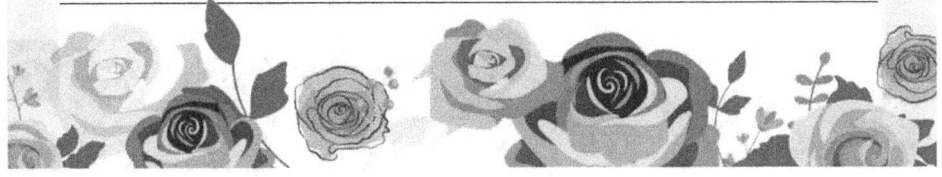

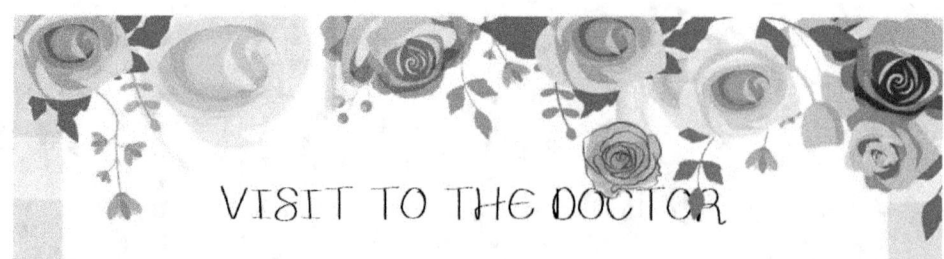

VISIT TO THE DOCTOR

Date		Date	
Doctor		Doctor	
Hospital or Clinic		Hospital or Clinic	
Reason for Visit		Reason for Visit	
Diasnosis		Diasnosis	
Doctor's Comment & Notes		Doctor,s Comment & Notes	
Follow Up		Follow Up	

Date		Date	
Doctor		Doctor	
Hospital or Clinic		Hospital or Clinic	
Reason for Visit		Reason for Visit	
Diasnosis		Diasnosis	
Doctor's Comment & Notes		Doctor's Comment & Notes	
Follow Up		Follow Up	

Notes:

_____

_____

_____

_____

_____

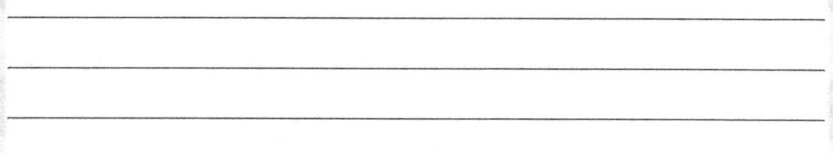

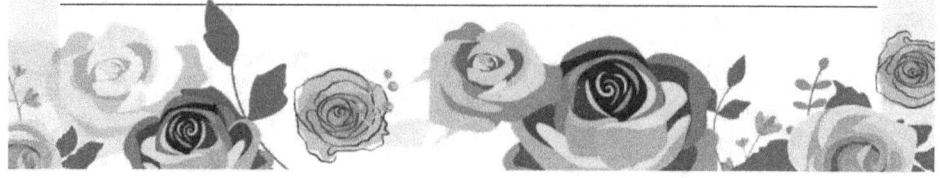

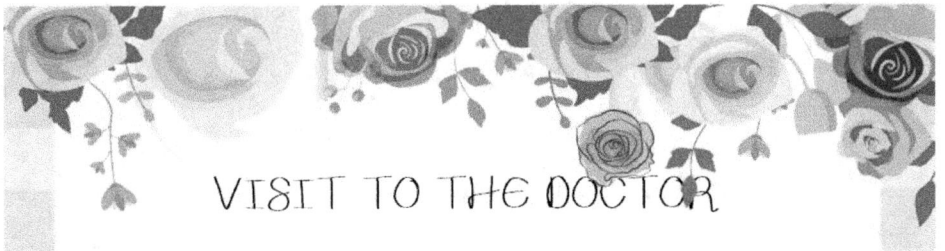

VISIT TO THE DOCTOR

Date	
Doctor	
Hospital or Clinic	
Reason for Visit	
Diasnosis	
Doctor's Comment & Notes	
Follow Up	

Date	
Doctor	
Hospital or Clinic	
Reason for Visit	
Diasnosis	
Doctor,s Comment & Notes	
Follow Up	

Date	
Doctor	
Hospital or Clinic	
Reason for Visit	
Diasnosis	
Doctor's Comment & Notes	
Follow Up	

Date	
Doctor	
Hospital or Clinic	
Reason for Visit	
Diasnosis	
Doctor's Comment & Notes	
Follow Up	

Notes:
_____

_____

_____

_____

_____

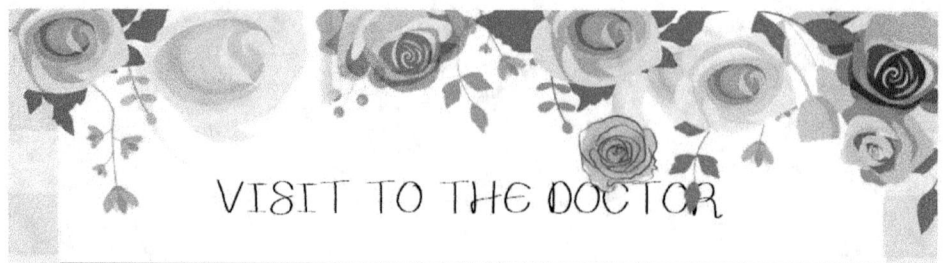

VISIT TO THE DOCTOR

Date	
Doctor	
Hospital or Clinic	
Reason for Visit	
Diasnosis	
Doctor's Comment & Notes	
Follow Up	

Date	
Doctor	
Hospital or Clinic	
Reason for Visit	
Diasnosis	
Doctor,s Comment & Notes	
Follow Up	

Date	
Doctor	
Hospital or Clinic	
Reason for Visit	
Diasnosis	
Doctor's Comment & Notes	
Follow Up	

Date	
Doctor	
Hospital or Clinic	
Reason for Visit	
Diasnosis	
Doctor's Comment & Notes	
Follow Up	

Notes:

_____

_____

_____

_____

_____

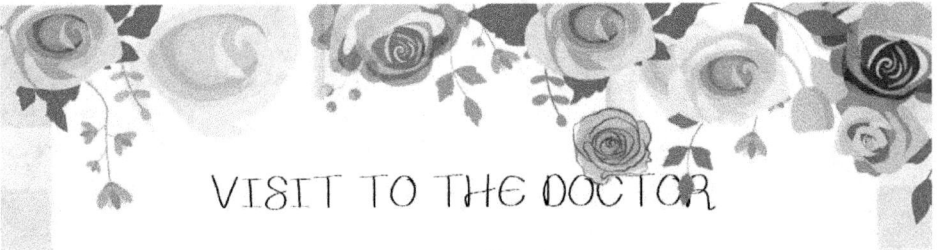

VISIT TO THE DOCTOR

Date	
Doctor	
Hospital or Clinic	
Reason for Visit	
Diasnosis	
Doctor's Comment & Notes	
Follow Up	

Date	
Doctor	
Hospital or Clinic	
Reason for Visit	
Diasnosis	
Doctor,s Comment & Notes	
Follow Up	

Date	
Doctor	
Hospital or Clinic	
Reason for Visit	
Diasnosis	
Doctor's Comment & Notes	
Follow Up	

Date	
Doctor	
Hospital or Clinic	
Reason for Visit	
Diasnosis	
Doctor's Comment & Notes	
Follow Up	

Notes:

_____

_____

_____

_____

_____

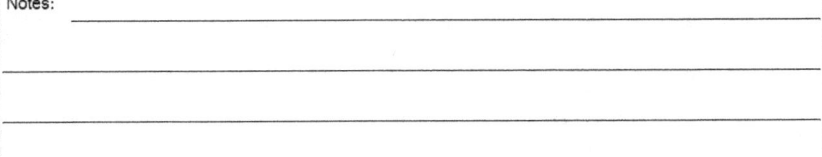

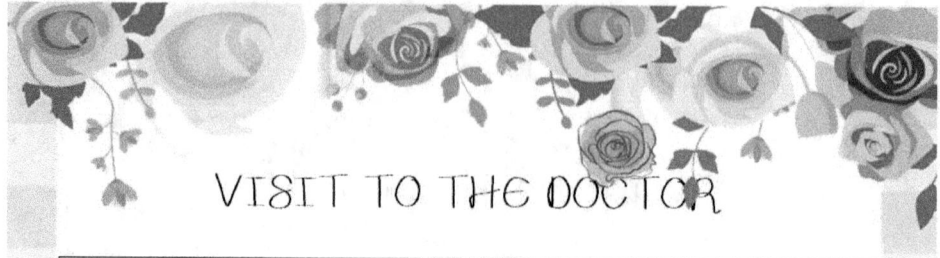

VISIT TO THE DOCTOR

Date	
Doctor	
Hospital or Clinic	
Reason for Visit	
Diasnosis	
Doctor's Comment & Notes	
Follow Up	

Date	
Doctor	
Hospital or Clinic	
Reason for Visit	
Diasnosis	
Doctor,s Comment & Notes	
Follow Up	

Date	
Doctor	
Hospital or Clinic	
Reason for Visit	
Diasnosis	
Doctor's Comment & Notes	
Follow Up	

Date	
Doctor	
Hospital or Clinic	
Reason for Visit	
Diasnosis	
Doctor's Comment & Notes	
Follow Up	

Notes:

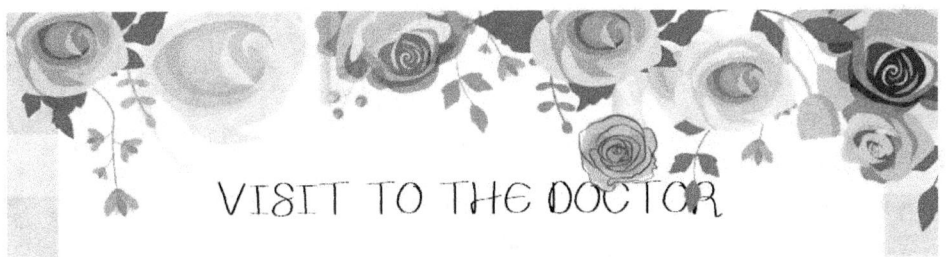

VISIT TO THE DOCTOR

Date	
Doctor	
Hospital or Clinic	
Reason for Visit	
Diasnosis	
Doctor's Comment & Notes	
Follow Up	

Date	
Doctor	
Hospital or Clinic	
Reason for Visit	
Diasnosis	
Doctor,s Comment & Notes	
Follow Up	

Date	
Doctor	
Hospital or Clinic	
Reason for Visit	
Diasnosis	
Doctor's Comment & Notes	
Follow Up	

Date	
Doctor	
Hospital or Clinic	
Reason for Visit	
Diasnosis	
Doctor's Comment & Notes	
Follow Up	

Notes: _____

_____

_____

_____

_____

_____

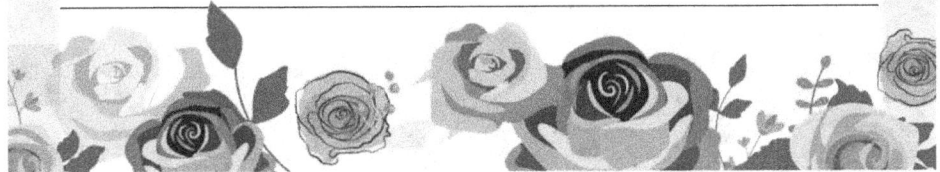

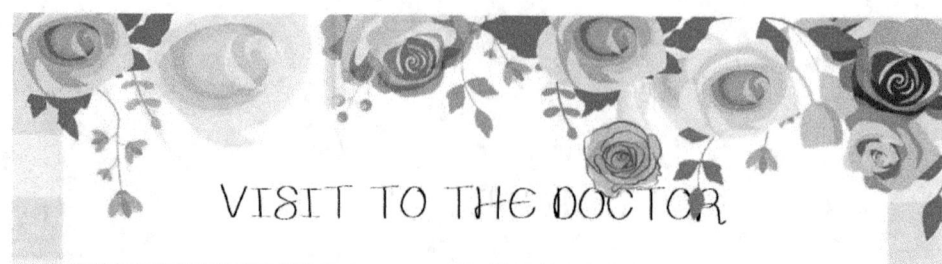

VISIT TO THE DOCTOR

Date	
Doctor	
Hospital or Clinic	
Reason for Visit	
Diasnosis	
Doctor's Comment & Notes	
Follow Up	

Date	
Doctor	
Hospital or Clinic	
Reason for Visit	
Diasnosis	
Doctor,s Comment & Notes	
Follow Up	

Date	
Doctor	
Hospital or Clinic	
Reason for Visit	
Diasnosis	
Doctor's Comment & Notes	
Follow Up	

Date	
Doctor	
Hospital or Clinic	
Reason for Visit	
Diasnosis	
Doctor's Comment & Notes	
Follow Up	

Notes:

_____

_____

_____

_____

_____

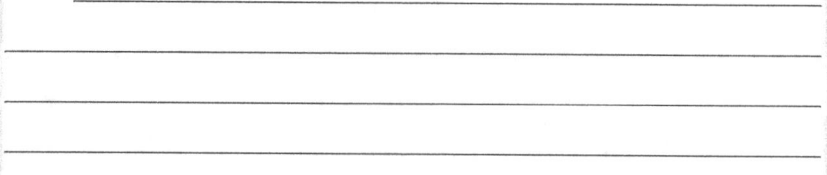

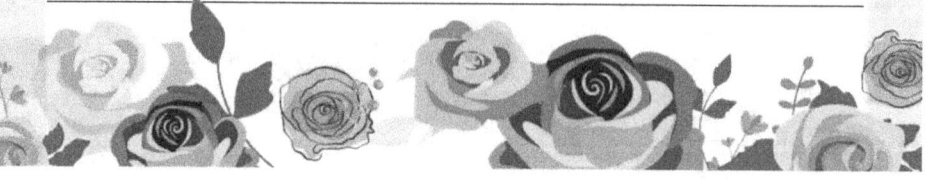

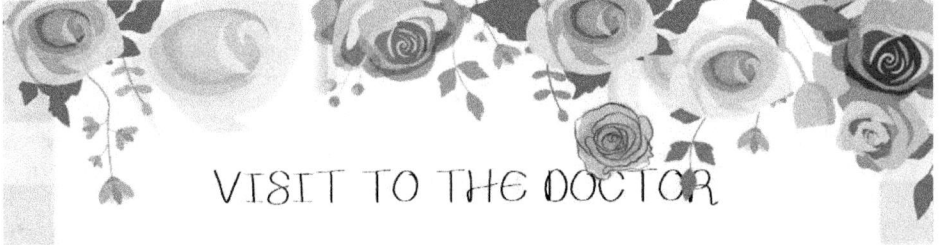

VISIT TO THE DOCTOR

Date	
Doctor	
Hospital or Clinic	
Reason for Visit	
Diasnosis	
Doctor's Comment & Notes	
Follow Up	

Date	
Doctor	
Hospital or Clinic	
Reason for Visit	
Diasnosis	
Doctor,s Comment & Notes	
Follow Up	

Date	
Doctor	
Hospital or Clinic	
Reason for Visit	
Diasnosis	
Doctor's Comment & Notes	
Follow Up	

Date	
Doctor	
Hospital or Clinic	
Reason for Visit	
Diasnosis	
Doctor's Comment & Notes	
Follow Up	

Notes:

_____

_____

_____

_____

_____

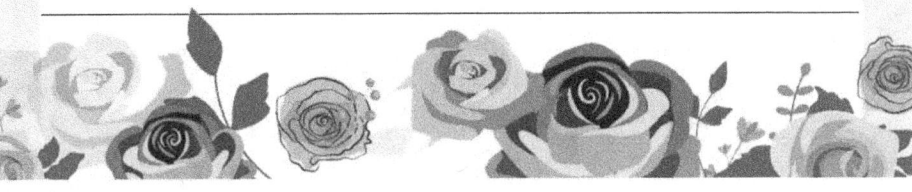

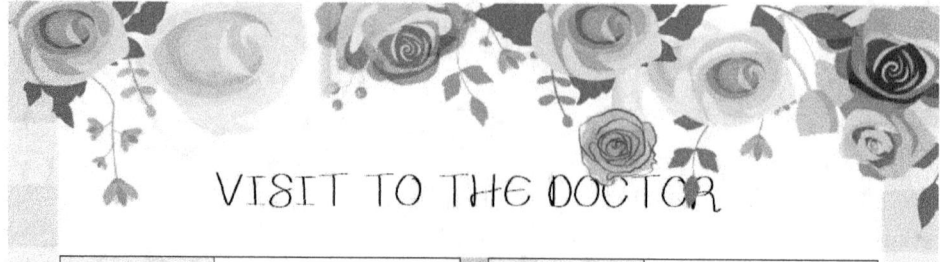

VISIT TO THE DOCTOR

Date	
Doctor	
Hospital or Clinic	
Reason for Visit	
Diasnosis	
Doctor's Comment & Notes	
Follow Up	

Date	
Doctor	
Hospital or Clinic	
Reason for Visit	
Diasnosis	
Doctor,s Comment & Notes	
Follow Up	

Date	
Doctor	
Hospital or Clinic	
Reason for Visit	
Diasnosis	
Doctor's Comment & Notes	
Follow Up	

Date	
Doctor	
Hospital or Clinic	
Reason for Visit	
Diasnosis	
Doctor's Comment & Notes	
Follow Up	

Notes:

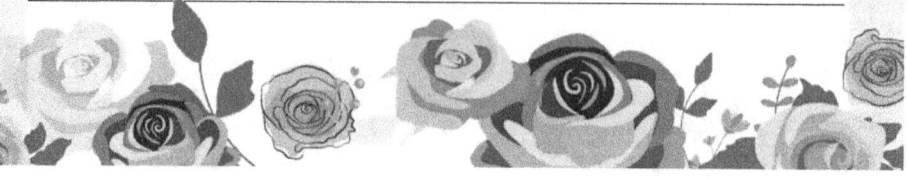

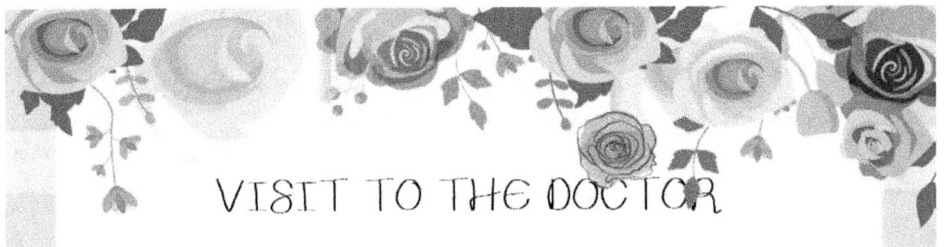

VISIT TO THE DOCTOR

Date	
Doctor	
Hospital or Clinic	
Reason for Visit	
Diasnosis	
Doctor's Comment & Notes	
Follow Up	

Date	
Doctor	
Hospital or Clinic	
Reason for Visit	
Diasnosis	
Doctor,s Comment & Notes	
Follow Up	

Date	
Doctor	
Hospital or Clinic	
Reason for Visit	
Diasnosis	
Doctor's Comment & Notes	
Follow Up	

Date	
Doctor	
Hospital or Clinic	
Reason for Visit	
Diasnosis	
Doctor's Comment & Notes	
Follow Up	

Notes:

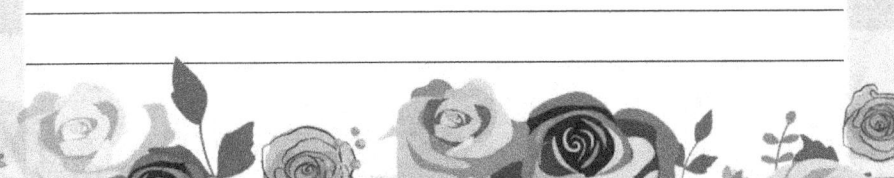

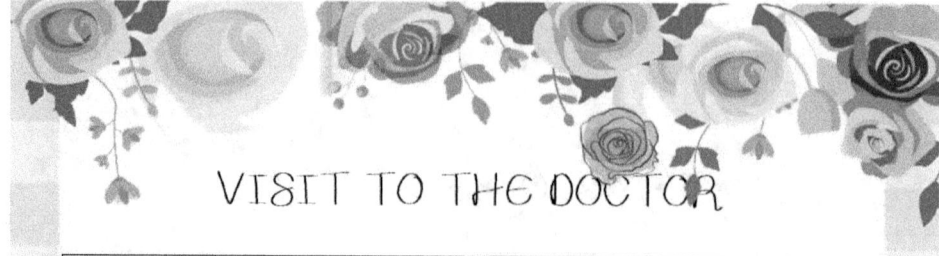

VISIT TO THE DOCTOR

Date			Date	
Doctor			Doctor	
Hospital or Clinic			Hospital or Clinic	
Reason for Visit			Reason for Visit	
Diasnosis			Diasnosis	
Doctor's Comment & Notes			Doctor,s Comment & Notes	
Follow Up			Follow Up	

Date			Date	
Doctor			Doctor	
Hospital or Clinic			Hospital or Clinic	
Reason for Visit			Reason for Visit	
Diasnosis			Diasnosis	
Doctor's Comment & Notes			Doctor's Comment & Notes	
Follow Up			Follow Up	

Notes:

_____

_____

_____

_____

_____

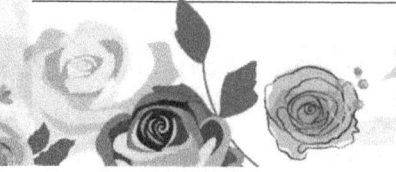

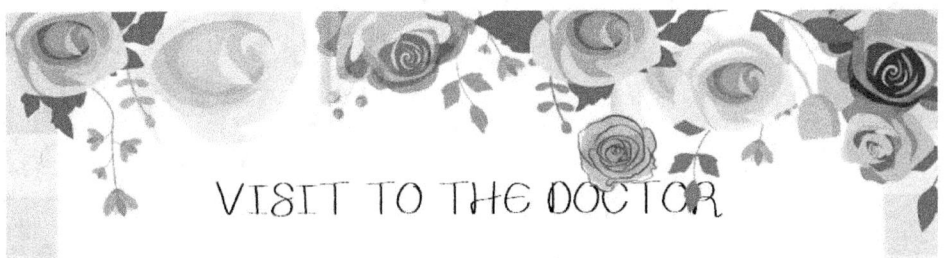

VISIT TO THE DOCTOR

Date	
Doctor	
Hospital or Clinic	
Reason for Visit	
Diasnosis	
Doctor's Comment & Notes	
Follow Up	

Date	
Doctor	
Hospital or Clinic	
Reason for Visit	
Diasnosis	
Doctor,s Comment & Notes	
Follow Up	

Date	
Doctor	
Hospital or Clinic	
Reason for Visit	
Diasnosis	
Doctor's Comment & Notes	
Follow Up	

Date	
Doctor	
Hospital or Clinic	
Reason for Visit	
Diasnosis	
Doctor's Comment & Notes	
Follow Up	

Notes:

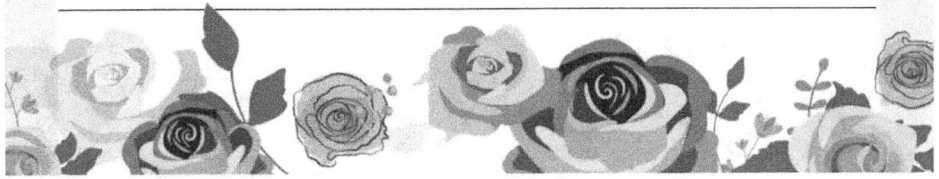

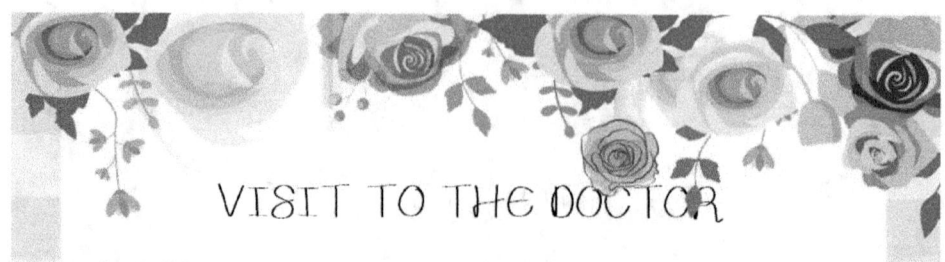

VISIT TO THE DOCTOR

Date	
Doctor	
Hospital or Clinic	
Reason for Visit	
Diasnosis	
Doctor's Comment & Notes	
Follow Up	

Date	
Doctor	
Hospital or Clinic	
Reason for Visit	
Diasnosis	
Doctor,s Comment & Notes	
Follow Up	

Date	
Doctor	
Hospital or Clinic	
Reason for Visit	
Diasnosis	
Doctor's Comment & Notes	
Follow Up	

Date	
Doctor	
Hospital or Clinic	
Reason for Visit	
Diasnosis	
Doctor's Comment & Notes	
Follow Up	

Notes:

_____

_____

_____

_____

_____

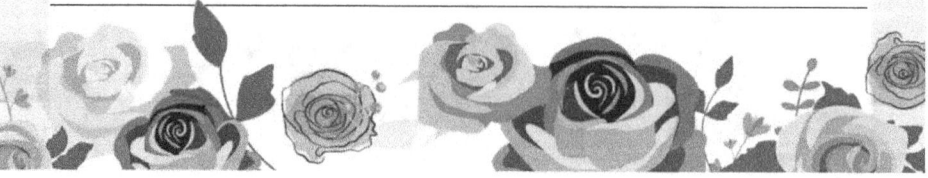

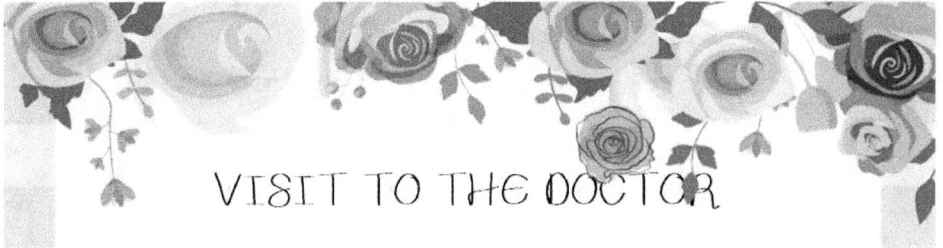

VISIT TO THE DOCTOR

Date	
Doctor	
Hospital or Clinic	
Reason for Visit	
Diasnosis	
Doctor's Comment & Notes	
Follow Up	

Date	
Doctor	
Hospital or Clinic	
Reason for Visit	
Diasnosis	
Doctor,s Comment & Notes	
Follow Up	

Date	
Doctor	
Hospital or Clinic	
Reason for Visit	
Diasnosis	
Doctor's Comment & Notes	
Follow Up	

Date	
Doctor	
Hospital or Clinic	
Reason for Visit	
Diasnosis	
Doctor's Comment & Notes	
Follow Up	

Notes: _____

_____

_____

_____

_____

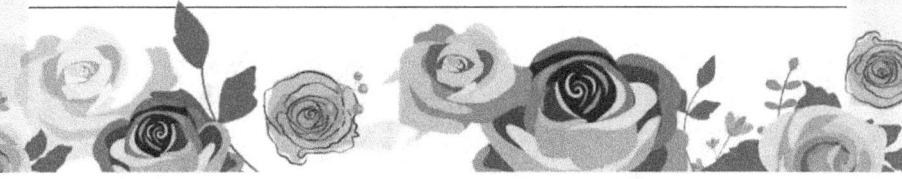

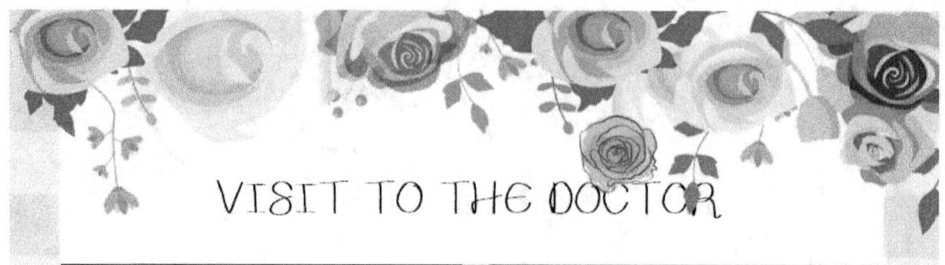

VISIT TO THE DOCTOR

Date	
Doctor	
Hospital or Clinic	
Reason for Visit	
Diasnosis	
Doctor's Comment & Notes	
Follow Up	

Date	
Doctor	
Hospital or Clinic	
Reason for Visit	
Diasnosis	
Doctor,s Comment & Notes	
Follow Up	

Date	
Doctor	
Hospital or Clinic	
Reason for Visit	
Diasnosis	
Doctor's Comment & Notes	
Follow Up	

Date	
Doctor	
Hospital or Clinic	
Reason for Visit	
Diasnosis	
Doctor's Comment & Notes	
Follow Up	

Notes:

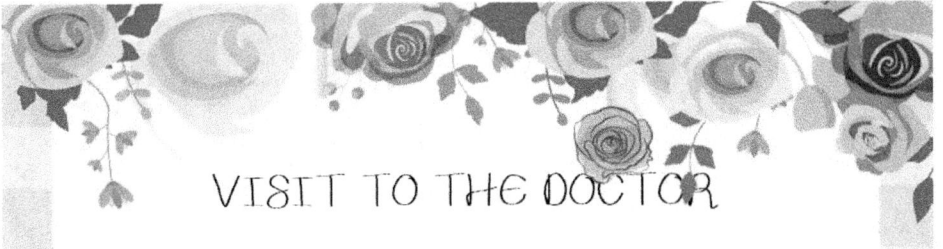

VISIT TO THE DOCTOR

Date		Date	
Doctor		Doctor	
Hospital or Clinic		Hospital or Clinic	
Reason for Visit		Reason for Visit	
Diasnosis		Diasnosis	
Doctor's Comment & Notes		Doctor,s Comment & Notes	
Follow Up		Follow Up	

Date		Date	
Doctor		Doctor	
Hospital or Clinic		Hospital or Clinic	
Reason for Visit		Reason for Visit	
Diasnosis		Diasnosis	
Doctor's Comment & Notes		Doctor's Comment & Notes	
Follow Up		Follow Up	

Notes:

_____

_____

_____

_____

_____

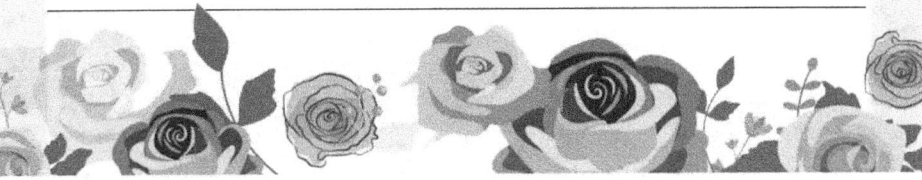

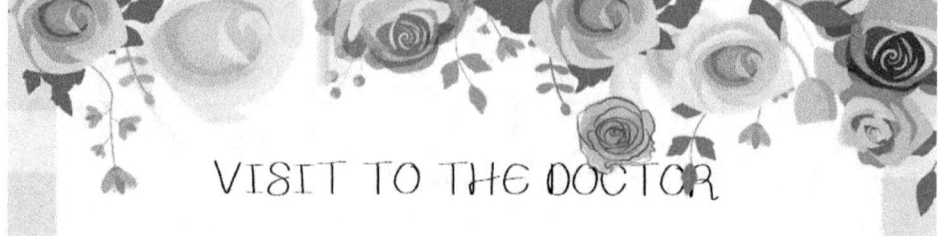

VISIT TO THE DOCTOR

Date	
Doctor	
Hospital or Clinic	
Reason for Visit	
Diasnosis	
Doctor's Comment & Notes	
Follow Up	

Date	
Doctor	
Hospital or Clinic	
Reason for Visit	
Diasnosis	
Doctor,s Comment & Notes	
Follow Up	

Date	
Doctor	
Hospital or Clinic	
Reason for Visit	
Diasnosis	
Doctor's Comment & Notes	
Follow Up	

Date	
Doctor	
Hospital or Clinic	
Reason for Visit	
Diasnosis	
Doctor's Comment & Notes	
Follow Up	

Notes:
_____
_____
_____
_____
_____
_____

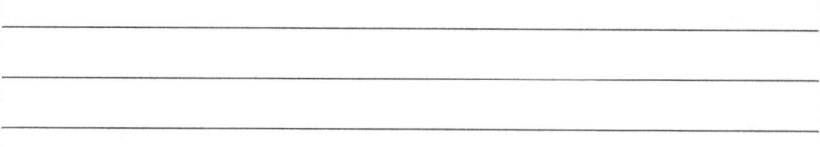
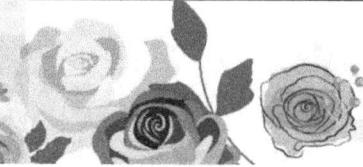

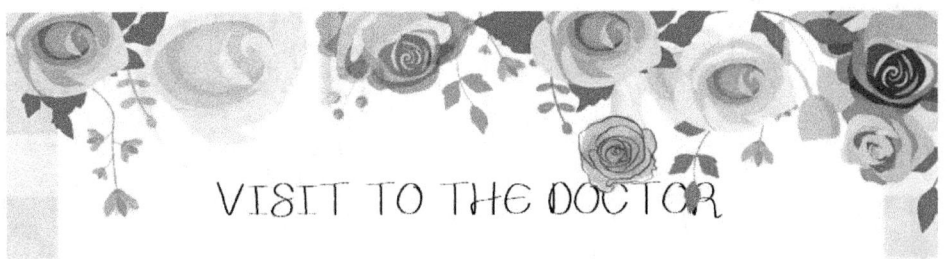

VISIT TO THE DOCTOR

Date	
Doctor	
Hospital or Clinic	
Reason for Visit	
Diasnosis	
Doctor's Comment & Notes	
Follow Up	

Date	
Doctor	
Hospital or Clinic	
Reason for Visit	
Diasnosis	
Doctor,s Comment & Notes	
Follow Up	

Date	
Doctor	
Hospital or Clinic	
Reason for Visit	
Diasnosis	
Doctor's Comment & Notes	
Follow Up	

Date	
Doctor	
Hospital or Clinic	
Reason for Visit	
Diasnosis	
Doctor's Comment & Notes	
Follow Up	

Notes: _____

_____

_____

_____

_____

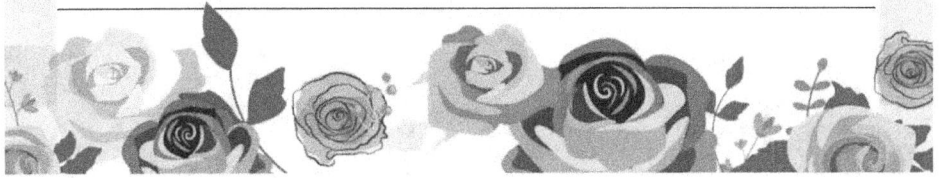

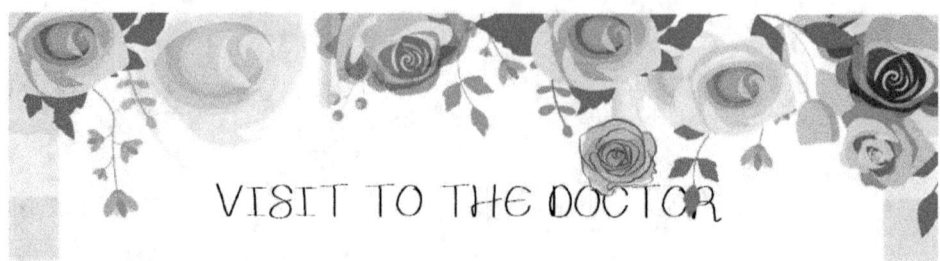

VISIT TO THE DOCTOR

Date		Date	
Doctor		Doctor	
Hospital or Clinic		Hospital or Clinic	
Reason for Visit		Reason for Visit	
Diasnosis		Diasnosis	
Doctor's Comment & Notes		Doctor,s Comment & Notes	
Follow Up		Follow Up	

Date		Date	
Doctor		Doctor	
Hospital or Clinic		Hospital or Clinic	
Reason for Visit		Reason for Visit	
Diasnosis		Diasnosis	
Doctor's Comment & Notes		Doctor's Comment & Notes	
Follow Up		Follow Up	

Notes:

_____

_____

_____

_____

_____

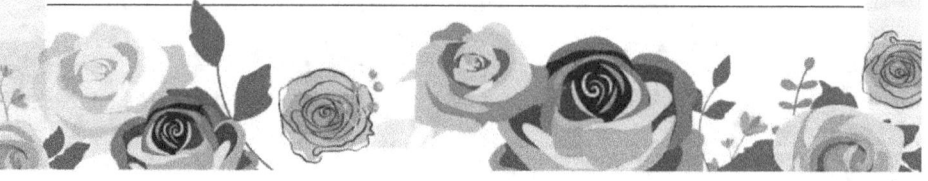

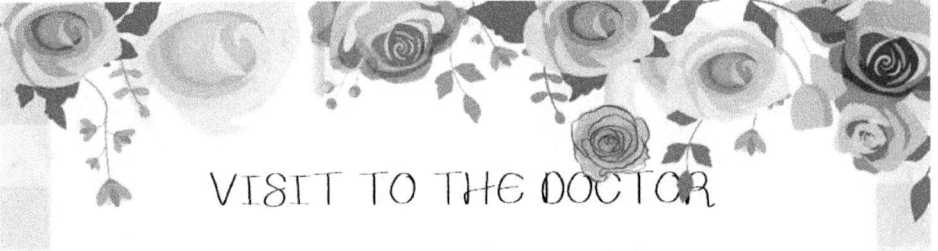

VISIT TO THE DOCTOR

Date	
Doctor	
Hospital or Clinic	
Reason for Visit	
Diasnosis	
Doctor's Comment & Notes	
Follow Up	

Date	
Doctor	
Hospital or Clinic	
Reason for Visit	
Diasnosis	
Doctor,s Comment & Notes	
Follow Up	

Date	
Doctor	
Hospital or Clinic	
Reason for Visit	
Diasnosis	
Doctor's Comment & Notes	
Follow Up	

Date	
Doctor	
Hospital or Clinic	
Reason for Visit	
Diasnosis	
Doctor's Comment & Notes	
Follow Up	

Notes:

_____

_____

_____

_____

_____

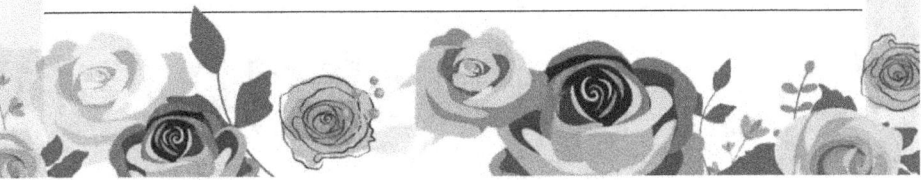

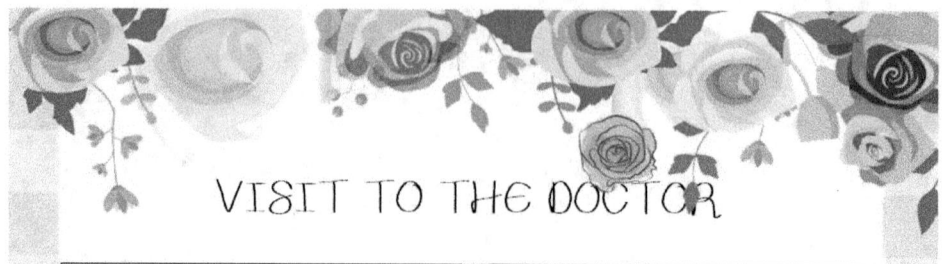

VISIT TO THE DOCTOR

Date		Date	
Doctor		Doctor	
Hospital or Clinic		Hospital or Clinic	
Reason for Visit		Reason for Visit	
Diasnosis		Diasnosis	
Doctor's Comment & Notes		Doctor,s Comment & Notes	
Follow Up		Follow Up	

Date		Date	
Doctor		Doctor	
Hospital or Clinic		Hospital or Clinic	
Reason for Visit		Reason for Visit	
Diasnosis		Diasnosis	
Doctor's Comment & Notes		Doctor's Comment & Notes	
Follow Up		Follow Up	

Notes:

_____

_____

_____

_____

_____

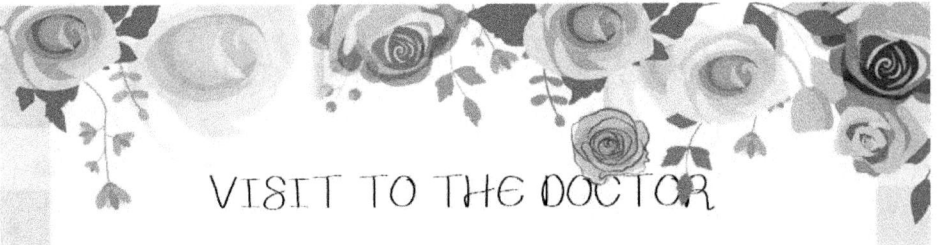

VISIT TO THE DOCTOR

Date	
Doctor	
Hospital or Clinic	
Reason for Visit	
Diasnosis	
Doctor's Comment & Notes	
Follow Up	

Date	
Doctor	
Hospital or Clinic	
Reason for Visit	
Diasnosis	
Doctor,s Comment & Notes	
Follow Up	

Date	
Doctor	
Hospital or Clinic	
Reason for Visit	
Diasnosis	
Doctor's Comment & Notes	
Follow Up	

Date	
Doctor	
Hospital or Clinic	
Reason for Visit	
Diasnosis	
Doctor's Comment & Notes	
Follow Up	

Notes:

_____

_____

_____

_____

_____

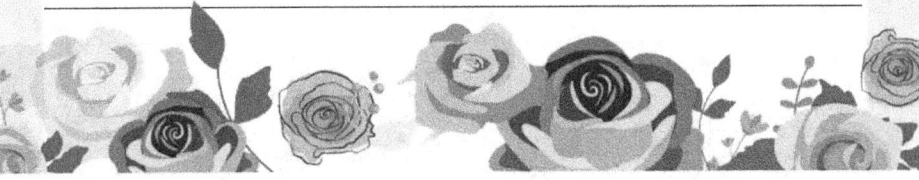

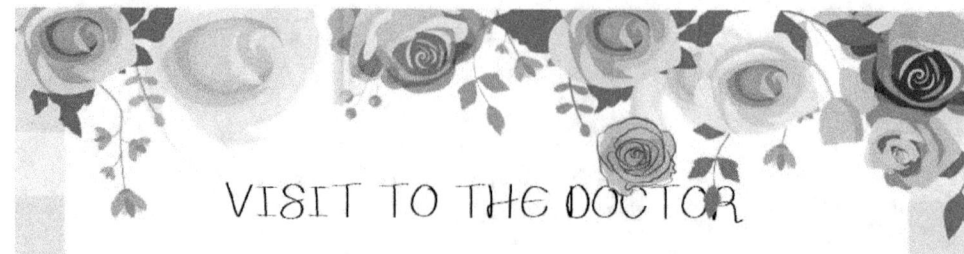

VISIT TO THE DOCTOR

Date	
Doctor	
Hospital or Clinic	
Reason for Visit	
Diasnosis	
Doctor's Comment & Notes	
Follow Up	

Date	
Doctor	
Hospital or Clinic	
Reason for Visit	
Diasnosis	
Doctor,s Comment & Notes	
Follow Up	

Date	
Doctor	
Hospital or Clinic	
Reason for Visit	
Diasnosis	
Doctor's Comment & Notes	
Follow Up	

Date	
Doctor	
Hospital or Clinic	
Reason for Visit	
Diasnosis	
Doctor's Comment & Notes	
Follow Up	

Notes:

_____

_____

_____

_____

_____

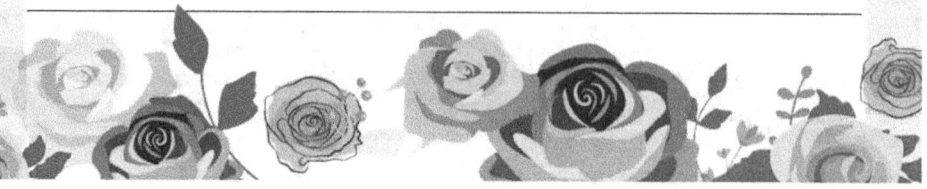

NOTES

NOTES

NOTES

NOTES

NOTES

NOTES

NOTES

NOTES

ISBN-13:978-1983832055
ISBN-10:1983832057